HIV/AIDS and the Stage: Politics and Performance in Neoliberal Times

REPRESENTATIONS: HEALTH, DISABILITY, CULTURE AND SOCIETY

Series Editor
Stuart Murray, University of Leeds

This series provides a ground-breaking and innovative selection of titles that showcase the newest interdisciplinary research on the cultural representations of health and disability in the contemporary social world. Bringing together both subjects and working methods from literary studies, film and cultural studies, medicine and sociology, 'Representations' is scholarly and accessible, addressed to researchers across a number of academic disciplines, and practitioners and members of the public with interests in issues of public health.

The key term in the series will be representations. Public interest in questions of health and disability has never been stronger, and as a consequence cultural forms across a range of media currently produce a never-ending stream of narratives and images that both reflect this interest and generate its forms. The crucial value of the series is that it brings the skilled study of cultural narratives and images to bear on such contemporary medical concerns. It offers and responds to new research paradigms that advance understanding at a scholarly level of the interaction between medicine, culture and society; it also has a strong commitment to public concerns surrounding such issues, and maintains a tone and point of address that seek to engage a general audience.

Other books in the series

Disabled Bodies in Early Modern Spanish Literature: Prostitutes, Aging Women and Saints
Encarnación Juárez-Almendros

Articulating Bodies: The Narrative Form of Disability and Illness in Victorian Fiction
Kylee-Anne Hingston

Disability, Literature, Genre: Representation and Affect in Contemporary Fiction
Ria Cheyne

Disability and the Posthuman: Bodies, Technology, and Cultural Futures
Stuart Murray

HIV/AIDS and the Stage

Politics and Performance in Neoliberal Times

Louisa Hann

LIVERPOOL UNIVERSITY PRESS

First published 2024 by
Liverpool University Press
4 Cambridge Street
Liverpool
L69 7ZU

British Library Cataloguing-in-Publication data
A British Library CIP record is available

ISBN 978-1-83553-759-6 hb

Typeset by Carnegie Book Production, Lancaster

Contents

Acknowledgements

This book was written in the months and years following my doctoral program – almost always (and increasingly) a precarious and hectic time for researchers in the arts and humanities. So it's well worth underlining the roles of the many who made it all possible. Firstly, I'd like to extend my gratitude to those who helped kickstart this book project in the months following my PhD. A short-term ECR Fellowship awarded by the Northern Network for Medical Humanities Research helped me eke out some time to put a proposal together and gather my thoughts. Alice Hall provided valuable mentorship and encouragement during this time, including feedback on my initial proposal. The team of editors at Liverpool University Press have also made the experience of publishing a first book a smooth and enjoyable one. Two anonymous reviewers delivered very generous and thoughtful feedback while helping rein in some of my more jarring rhetorical flourishes. Thanks also to all those at the University of Manchester who helped shape the PhD thesis upon which this book is based – notably my PhD supervisor David Alderson. My thesis examiners, Stephen Greer and Eithne Quinn, also provided helpful advice for developing the work following my viva.

Naturally, supportive friends and family also played a sizable role in getting my manuscript over the finishing line. Significant chunks of the book were written during coffee-fueled writing sessions with Jo Jones and Anirudha Dhanawade – long may they continue (and thanks to Folk café in Didsbury for hosting). José Saleiro Gomes and Stian Kristensen were fantastic pals to research and write my PhD alongside (and both continue to deliver unrivalled film recommendations). Mickey Cooper's daily WhatsApp messages and regular questioning about when this book will be published provided ample motivation during writing slumps, while weeknight dinners and reality TV sessions with Phil Watson offered light relief following long writing days. The same can be said for the countless hours whiled away with my many 'Garden Time' friends – despite the fact Manchester's weather means we rarely meet outdoors. Will Addy provided more reassurance and support than he probably realizes. And finally – thanks to my brother, Pat, and my parents, Dave and Jenny, for their unwavering love and support.

Introduction: Theater, HIV/AIDS, and the Neoliberal Revolution

The history of the HIV/AIDS pandemic provides an exemplary lesson in the failures of neoliberal capitalism. Up to 48.6 million people worldwide are estimated to have died of HIV/AIDS-related complications since the pandemic's inception (World Health Organization 2020), a death toll that raises urgent questions about the extent to which society's primary distributive system has equipped us with the resources, technologies, and systems of care required to minimize the virus's threat to life and wellbeing. Unsurprisingly, perhaps, the evidence does not point in capitalism's favor. A confluence of its essential mechanisms – including an insatiable 'growth' or profit imperative, a disproportionate reliance on racialized and otherwise subjugated people to generate such profit, and the creation of surplus populations cast as less deserving of health and social care – has allowed HIV/AIDS to spread through marginalized constituencies the world over (although primarily in the Global South). First brought to the attention of world leaders and pharmaceutical companies in the early 1980s, initial responses to the HIV/AIDS pandemic were sluggish, dismissive, and hindered by stigma. Most famously, perhaps, US President Ronald Reagan avoided the public mention of AIDS until 1985, by which point the country's Centers for Disease Control and Prevention (CDC) had identified all major transmission routes (Bennington-Castro 2020). As a result of such negligence, well over a decade passed before effective drugs were developed, access to which remains patchy for those populations neoliberalism works to impoverish.

In some ways, the pandemic's trajectory and epidemiological structure parallels those of other viral health threats of such magnitude under our current socio-economic system. As Steven W. Thrasher explains in his theorization of the 'viral underclass', viruses like HIV and SARS-CoV-2 (the virus that causes COVID-19) shine a bright light on societal inequities. Such crises catalyze neoliberalism's immiserating function, pushing more people into poverty while shoring up riches for the wealthy. Within months of the start of the COVID-19 pandemic and the imposition of social distancing measures (including 'lockdowns') in the US, 'more than 40 million people had lost their jobs (ironically, including nearly a million and a half health care workers). Meanwhile, approximately 27 million people lost their health insurance' (Thrasher 2022). The fact that capitalism poses more corporeal threats to the poor and marginalized is surely as stark as ever in an age of COVID-19, reminding us of the ways in which HIV disproportionately affects similarly classed constituencies. However, the relation of HIV/AIDS to the contemporary political economy contains unique specificities by dint of its pathogenetic and epidemiological characteristics. Unlike many of the other viruses to have erupted over the past few decades – including Ebola, SARS-CoV-2, and a host of other coronaviruses – HIV usually spreads via the direct transfer of blood, semen, and rectal and vaginal fluids, as well as from mother to child during pregnancy. It is more prevalent in men who have sex with men, with anal sex representing one of the ways through which transmission commonly occurs. People who inject drugs are also disproportionately susceptible to HIV if they share needles containing traces of other people's blood. As a result, the constituencies affected by HIV/AIDS are even more likely to be those which neoliberal capitalism works to subjugate and marginalize – the queer, the poor, the racialized, and the criminalized.

Running alongside histories detailing the catastrophic effects of HIV/AIDS on certain 'risk groups' are those concerning the counterhegemonic pushback against institutional, corporate, and state neglect. The US spawned some of the world's best-known grassroots movements to tackle HIV/AIDS – most notably the AIDS Coalition to Unleash Power (ACT UP), which garnered headlines for its confrontational tactics challenging powerful state and corporate institutions. Often bound up with these activist groups were artistic and cultural movements highlighting the injustices affecting people living with HIV. Playwrights and performance artists were especially prolific during the early years of the crisis, as frequently revived hits including Larry Kramer's *The Normal Heart* (1985), Tony Kushner's *Angels in America* (1991), Paul Rudnick's *Jeffrey* (1993), and Jonathan Larson's *Rent* (1996) were premiered in New York and other major cities.

Beyond the Broadway hits, lesser-known plays graced smaller theaters and countercultural stages across the country. Spurred on by fringe and amateur theater's relatively low cost and accessibility (compared with, say, the film, television, and literary worlds), activists and like-minded comrades produced a range of plays aimed at galvanizing support for people with HIV fighting oppressive forces, and educating audiences about the everyday realities of HIV/AIDS. To some extent, then, the stage delivered political opportunities to speak out against state and societal neglect and demonization.

At the same time, however, neoliberal hegemony was already well on its way to capturing both the organizational structures of theatrical institutions and the attitudes of their resident playwrights. While the intellectual, political, and material histories of neoliberalism are complex and hotly contested, many recognize Margaret Thatcher and Ronald Reagan as pioneering its first wave around the late 1970s and early 1980s (Steger and Roy 2010, 21). Grappling to protect the capitalist order as Keynesianism faltered, both figures implemented policy changes that shored up the power of finance capital, encouraged privatization, slashed public expenditure, and ultimately produced 'a world where competition is the primary virtue, and solidarity a sign of weakness' (Mirowski 2014, 92). For theaters, this socio-economic shift saw state funding dwindle and artists increasingly subjected to competitive pressures and 'impact' requirements designed to identify the most profitable work – hardly fertile ground for experimental or counterhegemonic playwriting.

While the 2020s represent particularly bleak times for the creatively inclined, the effects of neoliberalization were already reverberating throughout the theater world by the turn of the millennium. As Maria M. Delgado and Caridad Svich emphasize in their pessimistic volume, *Theatre in Crisis? Performance Manifestos for a New Century* (2002), 'there are fewer forums for oppositional voices to be heard in a global economy that is eradicating difference in favour of a McSociety built in the celebration of the common dollar', while 'cuts in funding have radically affected the types of plays being written, as the epic play has largely been abandoned in favour of small cast texts which present fewer challenges on dwindling company budgets' (Delgado and Svich 2002, 7). As we will see, such a hostile economic landscape has compelled theater makers to forge highly precarious funding models, while warping and shaping attitudes toward public health, queer politics, HIV prevention, and, by extension, the content of HIV/AIDS plays.

This book will assess these intertwined – sometimes countervailing – phenomena to examine how the stage has been able to operate as a counterhegemonic space for constituencies grappling with HIV's many corporeal and social effects. I will home in on work produced in the Global North states most responsible for imposing neoliberalism as a dominant organizing logic on the rest of our interconnected world – not to perpetuate the historical sidelining of the Global South in HIV/AIDS scholarship, but to understand capitalism's role in popularizing some of the most acclaimed HIV/AIDS plays to date, problematize certain orthodoxies of contemporary HIV/AIDS scholarship, and uncover the reasons why some (indeed, most) constituencies affected by HIV/AIDS are so often overlooked by playwrights and performers. As well as populations in the Global South, such overlooked constituencies include women and racialized and otherwise marginalized groups largely shut out of a theatrical genre dominated by a white, gay, male subject.[1]

A significant proportion of the plays I will examine have emerged from the US – far and away the state most affected by HIV/AIDS in the Global North. To provide some sense of scale, more New Yorkers have died of AIDS since the beginning of the epidemic than the total number of AIDS deaths in Spain, Italy, the Netherlands, and Switzerland combined (Hobbes 2014). The virus also hit major US cities earlier and more forcefully than European metropolises, with 451 AIDS deaths recorded in the US in 1982, compared to only five in the UK (Hobbes 2014). While the reasons behind such disparities are complex and impossible to disentwine, the deep inequalities that characterize the world's largest economy have inevitably played a role in its (mis)handling of HIV/AIDS and, indeed, its artists' relationship with – and ability to push back against – hegemonic structures. As journalist Michael Hobbes notes, 'No health care system in the world has solved the problem of AIDS. The United Kingdom and Germany have gaps in their cascades, too. They struggle to control costs and reach marginalized populations the same as the States. They just have less margin to reach' (Hobbes 2014). While no collection of case studies will ever do justice to the breadth and diversity of HIV/AIDS theater as a heuristic and porous descriptor, my selection of case studies is designed to represent a variety of tendencies that emerge out of a

1 I refer to a broad (if imperfectly defined) 'HIV/AIDS genre' throughout this book, using this catch-all term to describe a group of plays and performance works that center HIV/AIDS as a key theme or political motivator. While no term can be deployed unproblematically in a study of this type, I believe this collective heuristic best describes the objects of study, linked as they are by common artistic forms, themes, concerns, and terms of debate.

capitalistic world. As such, I draw freely on plays from Global North states other than the US – most notably the UK – to illustrate neoliberal capture and resistance across global hegemons.[2]

Of course, there are significant differences across European and US contexts in terms of how people experienced and continue to experience HIV/AIDS. Writing in 1987, Simon Watney carefully examined how such social and cultural differences influenced the trajectory of HIV/AIDS in both the UK and the US in *Policing Desire: Pornography, AIDS and the Media*. While queer-identified people were firmly sidelined by hegemonic culture in the UK, Watney identified greater scope for identificatory and affective community building among its marginalized constituencies compared to those in the US. He notes:

> American gay culture has conspicuously failed to develop the types of collectivist institutions, organised neither for profit nor for sexual exploitation, which abound in Britain in the form of co-operatively owned cafes, discos, information switchboard services, legal organisations and publishing houses, as well as a flourishing tradition of independent gay theatre, pop music, film, poetry, and fiction, which is clearly at odds with dominant cultural values and institutions. For this there is little or no equivalent in the United States, where collectivism appears decidedly un-American. (Watney 1997, 15)

Some of my chosen American texts poke holes in this thesis. Countercultural performers such as Tim Miller turned small theatrical venues into spaces where queer kinship and consciousness raising could thrive, while provocateur Reza Abdoh led theater company Dar a Luz, an unapologetically queer outfit that member Sabrina Artel describes as a kind of 'family' united in its aims to shock the American

2 Beyond the thematic and contextual criteria established to conduct this study, it is worth acknowledging that material limitations have also shaped what works I have included or overlooked in this book. Much of this work is based on my PhD thesis. While I had some access to funding for archival research, travel, and theater tickets during my doctoral program, this funding was limited. I also significantly reworked and added new chapters to improve upon my original thesis – work that was (for the most part) undertaken while untethered from an institution, curbing my ability to access more obscure works. As such, this book inevitably omits certain works that might have emerged within more radical or underground contexts. I aim for my focus on more mainstream and easily accessible HIV/AIDS theater to provide the basis for further materialist discussion of HIV/AIDS theater in neoliberal (or, indeed, post-neoliberal) times.

public into understanding the violence hegemonic culture inflicts on the downtrodden and marginalized (Artel 1995, 72). However, there is compelling evidence that the enduring popularity of queer theater groups and co-creative collectives in the UK might reflect broader cultural differences.

Gay Sweatshop is one of the most notable examples, a radical theater collective established in 1974 with the aim of enlightening a broad public about the discrimination gay people faced, while debunking flagrant misrepresentations regularly published by reactionary media outlets. Gay Sweatshop was responsible for staging Andy Kirby's *Compromised Immunity* (1986), often celebrated as one of the UK's first AIDS plays and an antidote to rampant homophobia in its direct critiques of stereotypes surrounding gay men and people diagnosed with HIV. Other prominent institutions include Duckie, a collective that brought queer performance art and raucous club nights to London's Royal Vauxhall Tavern for over two decades, queer festivals Outburst Arts and Homotopia, and a peppering of long-running queer theaters across the UK's major cities.

Considering such differences in conjunction with the fact that US citizens were subject to a more punitive and marketized healthcare landscape and poorer access to welfare provisions, it becomes clear HIV/AIDS playwrights have had to navigate different obstacles, social attitudes, and institutional demands across countries. Where possible and relevant, therefore, I will situate performance works in their historical and political contexts. That being said, neoliberal dynamics seep across borders and, in many cases, are exported by hegemonic states to those with less power and global influence. For example, while the UK's National Health Service represents a lifeline of which the average American can only dream, decades of neoliberal governance have permitted privatization to infect much of the institution – a phenomenon linked to reduced quality of care and increased patient deaths (Mahase 2022). As such, many of the conclusions drawn in this study might be applied across regional and historical contexts. By highlighting how the HIV/AIDS theater genre has both fought and capitulated to capitalism's most disenfranchising tendencies, the coming chapters will reveal how capitalism's organizing principles present significant barriers to ameliorating the HIV/AIDS pandemic. Before we examine the ins and outs of the theater landscape, however, I will provide fundamental context about how neoliberalism has determined the global course of the pandemic so far.

A brief history of HIV/AIDS under neoliberalism

We begin our story in the US – a decisive actor in both the financialization of the world economy and the consolidation of 'commonsensical' neoliberal values as the Soviet Union disintegrated and the vestiges of non-capitalist society largely flittered away. When President Reagan took office in 1981, he inherited an economy plagued by high inflation, economic contraction, and high unemployment – a situation he vowed to fix via deregulatory programs that reduced the federal tax rate, significantly restricted federal expenditure, and disarmed regulatory bodies in a bid to reignite growth (Reagan 1981). Such a program reflects devotion to a certain aspect of neoliberalism that, as Jeremy Gilbert explains, valorizes 'deliberate intervention by government in order to encourage particular types of entrepreneurial, competitive, and commercial behaviour in citizens', grounded in the belief that self-interest is 'the only motive force in human life' and competition 'the most efficient and socially beneficial way for that force to express itself' (Gilbert 2013, 9).

In other words, Reaganite programs planted the seeds for a form of neoliberalism to which I will consistently return in this book. Encompassing a set of common-sense principles first articulated in what Manfred Steger and Ravi Roy term 'first-wave neoliberalism' during the Reagan and Thatcher years, neoliberalism centered around the notion that individual freedoms could be secured through governmental facilitation of free markets, reflecting a 'geopolitical imperative to stop the spread of communism and socialist developmentalism in the Third World' (Steger and Roy 2010, 47). Although neoliberalism has altered to accommodate a changing political landscape, its core buttressing of extreme individualism has remained constant, naturalizing commercialism and competitiveness to the extent that they now permeate almost every aspect of a person's quotidian experience. Following this doctrine, competition enriches the whole of society by promoting productivity and growth, while encouraging those in possession of capital to invest in further money-making schemes that eventually – supposedly – benefit workers' pay packets.

While the trickle-down model Reagan instituted might not have revealed the catastrophic scale of its shortcomings (or spuriousness) by the 1980s, his restriction of federal expenditure had severe implications for those most reliant on welfare provisions. As domestic policies further immiserated the poorest subsections of society, the Reagan administration ginned up consent for such policies by restricting the potential for solidarity, quelling dissent, and uniting America's right wing. The ruling class alienated sections of the wider citizenry from one another by perpetuating stigmatizing narratives that threw the moral fabric of racialized, queer, and otherwise subaltern groups into question – what Ange-Marie Hancock coined the 'politics of disgust' (Hancock 2004). Young (primarily Black) single mothers, for example, were demonized as 'welfare queens' living in relative luxury while freeloading off the state – a pathologizing stereotype 'shaped by inegalitarian traditions of racism, sexism, and classism from the dark side of an American political culture of freedom and rugged individualism' (Hancock 2004, 26). As well as being considered a drain on federal budgets, the unmarried 'welfare queen' threatened capitalism's reliance on the family unit as the key sphere within which (unwaged) social reproduction could take place. As such, maintaining hegemonic dominance through what Stuart Hall termed 'the long march of the Neo-liberal Revolution' (Hall 2011, 705) required the neoliberals in power to convince, coerce, and force women and minority constituencies to pursue social relations that served the needs of capital.

Another constituency that threatened the American right wing's competitive, alienated, family-oriented social order was the queer or LGBTQ+ community. Having gained several civil rights wins during the 1970s, the queer-identified saw the dawn of neoliberal rule reinvigorate old phobias that threatened their lives and livelihoods. As Reagan cozied up to America's evangelical right wing, groups such as the so-called Moral Majority – a political organization extolling the virtues of 'traditional' family life – gained public exposure. At the same time, the AIDS pandemic threw fuel onto the fire. On July 3, 1981 – mere months after Reagan's inauguration – *The New York Times* published an article with the headline 'Rare Cancer Seen in 41 Homosexuals', explaining:

> The cause of the outbreak is unknown, and there is as yet no evidence of contagion. But the doctors who have made the diagnoses, mostly in New York City and the San Francisco Bay area, are alerting other physicians who treat large numbers of homosexual men to the problem in an effort to help identify more cases and to reduce the delay in offering chemotherapy treatment. (Altman 1981)

At this point, scientists were unaware of the disease's etiology, or even whether patients' symptoms were certainly linked. However, the gay men who first presented with signs of AIDS-related complications were quickly heralded as evidence of God's wrath against same-sex relations and supposedly wayward lifestyles by far-right ideologues.

In fact, 'America was typologically configured as both Sodom and Ancient Greece, and homosexuality or even only tolerance of homosexuality leads it along the "road to ruin," thus simultaneously constructing a crisis and demonizing homosexuals' (Long 2005, 8). As we will explore later in this book, factions of the right with considerable influence and power cast the onset of the AIDS pandemic as a millenarian rupture in which the 'deviant' or 'sinful' members of society would meet their punishment, leaving those remaining to enjoy the fruits of a phantasmatic American dream contingent on the protection of a heteronorm grounded in the sanctity of the nuclear family.

Cold War paranoia and residual McCarthyite tendencies were deeply embedded within this evangelical, homophobic, and ruthlessly capitalistic cosmology. As Cindy Patton noted in 1985, 'Even today some rightist groups claim that homosexuality and even AIDS is a communist plot, despite the fact that communist countries and parties have generally been hostile toward homosexuality' (Patton 1985, 88). With various liberatory movements – most notably the gay and lesbian rights movement – having gained ground in the later decades of the twentieth century, right-wing groups and Republican politicians were primed to engage in so-called 'culture wars' against queer and otherwise minoritized groups. In so doing, they strove to salvage the more 'traditional' familial forms of earlier Fordist capitalism that supplied the socially necessary forms of unwaged domestic labor required to uphold sustained industrial growth. As part of this project, 'communism and faggotry were well established as threats to US security. Both were assaults from within US culture – infiltration by people who didn't look different to the untrained eye' (Patton 1985, 88). As AIDS became more dominant in the public consciousness, the right conceptualized its various physical symptoms as warning signs through which to identify the enemy within.

Perhaps inevitably, the dehumanization involved in painting people with HIV and the queer-identified as national threats was accompanied by particularly egregious examples of homophobia, xenophobia, and racism. As John-Manuel Andriote explains in a history of the epidemic in the US, Reagan

> suggested at a White House meeting [in 1986] that Libyan dictator Moamar Gadhafi, rumoured to enjoy dressing in drag, should be sent to San Francisco because "he likes to dress up so much". Secretary of State George Schultz diplomatically added, "Why don't we give him AIDS?" As fear gripped the nation, and although thousands of Americans were

> dead from AIDS, the epidemic was treated as a sick joke at the White House. (Andriote 1999, 141–2)

Such cruelty was not limited to rhetoric. For example, on top of the administration's outright refusal to even mention HIV/AIDS until 1985, the Justice Department decided in 1986 to legalize the firing of employees on the basis of an official – or even rumored – AIDS diagnosis (Andriote 1999, 140). Such legislation inevitably compounded the suffering of those with AIDS diagnoses, as well as their friends and loved ones. Material support and care services were also markedly thin on the ground. While some people with HIV/AIDS benefited from local, state-funded AIDS services, thousands of HIV-positive people in New York were left to fend for themselves by Democratic mayor Ed Koch (Andriote 1999, 89).

As a result of state neglect, marginalized communities started organizing mutual aid and direct actions among themselves, as well as reading up on the latest scientific literature to support the medical care of those with HIV diagnoses. The most notable grassroots movement to emerge in the US was ACT UP, whose confrontational direct actions quickly hit the headlines on mainstream news outlets and television channels throughout the country. One of the most widely documented actions was 'Seize Control of the FDA' on October 11, 1988, in which around 1,500 ACT UP members attempted to occupy the Food and Drug Administration (FDA) to demand shorter drug approval processes, improved ethical standards for clinical trials, financial support for experimental drug therapies, and better support for community groups helping keep people with HIV/AIDS alive (Crimp 2011). As well as plastering the FDA building with ACT UP banners and staging a mock 'trial' of those deemed responsible for state neglect, movement members used their media savvy and professional connections to disseminate their message as widely as possible. As ACT UP member Douglas Crimp noted, the organization went out of their way to generate press coverage surrounding the FDA action. As well as sending a detailed press kit that sold the event 'almost like a Hollywood movie', ACT UP conducted hundreds of phone calls to the press and scheduled media appearances around the country. As a result, 'the media were not only there to get the story, they knew what that story was, and they reported it with a degree of accuracy and sympathy that is, to say the least, unusual' (Crimp 2011). The event's wide publicization and impact on public consciousness forced the FDA to grant at least some of ACT UP's high-profile members greater attention and respect. As Sarah Schulman has noted, drug approval standards improved, and the FDA was suddenly amenable to activists' demands. Indeed, the 'demonstration was a really important piece in forcing the agency to realize they had to deal with ACT UP in a way that was different from how they were used to dealing with consumers' (Schulman 2021a, 133).

Perhaps unsurprisingly, strategic decisions surrounding the movement's relationships with mainstream media outlets, pharmaceutical companies, and federal agencies were highly contested. Details of ACT UP's internal disputes are well documented in Jim Hubbard and Sarah Schulman's ACT UP Oral History Project (Harvard College Library) – a rich archive of interviews with 187 ACT UP members – as well as documentary films such as Hubbard's *United in Anger* (2012) and a vast body of historical and political scholarship on the group, to which Schulman has contributed extensively. As she notes in recent work, the activity of ACT UP's Treatment and Data Committee (T&D) – who boasted medical expertise and held meetings with powerful corporate entities and state functionaries – caused consternation among members with less access to power. Tracy Morgan, for example, who spent years advocating for the lives of women with AIDS, 'saw the mostly male T&D advancing their treatment agenda through their relationships with the government, won by mass actions put on by the entire organization at the FDA and NIH [National Institutes of Health]' (Schulman 2021a, 583). In moving away from ACT UP's on-the-ground organizing to occupy seats in powerful places, T&D were believed to have pandered to the exclusionary logics of corporations and wider capitalistic society – an ideological rift that contributed at least in part to ACT UP's eventual splintering.

One of the more recent studies to have examined ACT UP's history from a fresh angle is Beatrice Adler-Bolton and Artie Vierkant's *Health Communism* (2022), which details some of the impossible decisions marginalized groups face in supporting individual members while holding capitalism's institutions to account. The pair cite T&D's race to find a cure and consequent willingness to collude with the medical-industrial complex as exemplifying the power of capitalism's dehumanizing logics to immiserate and overlook the most marginalized in society. Adopting a broadly Marxist framework, they argue that healthcare under capitalism is conceptualized as a tool through which to organize the 'healthy', productive citizenry and the 'surplus' populations too sick, debilitated, or 'undesirable' to exploit for profit. Those considered 'surplus' are cast as disposable and, therefore, a drain on social welfare systems. In debates about public spending, the fundamental question therefore becomes: 'In what ways are their lives social *burdens*, and what is to be done to empirically separate the "deserving" (a burden in society's interest to take on) from the "undeserving" (an *irredeemable* burden)?' (Adler-Bolton and Vierkant 2022, 21, emphasis in original). Although highly effective drugs started entering the market in the mid-1990s, in part due to ACT UP's tireless work, they largely ended up in the bodies of white, middle-class Americans, to the exclusion of Black, Indigenous, and poor communities. While capitalism's distributive tendencies remained intact, the possibility of equitable outcomes for the most marginalized US citizens with HIV/AIDS remained remote.

Of course, the consequences of US inaction were not anomalous or contained within the country's borders, as American firms and state institutions governed a significant portion of the pharmaceutical industry upon which the world continues to rely. In fact, the immiseration experienced in the US was replicated and amplified in the Global South – a tendency reflective of wider geopolitical relations. On the one hand, pharmaceutical companies' abilities to gouge prices and protect their so-called intellectual property left many regions without the tools necessary to quell infection rates. When anti-retroviral drugs were first introduced, they were patented at $15,000 per yearly regimen, and generic pharmaceutical companies were banned from producing the same drugs, despite being able to do so at a fraction of the price. It was not until 2003 that the World Trade Organization (WTO) allowed southern African nations to import generic drugs, by which point millions of people in the region were infected with HIV (Hickel 2013). While such statistics are alarming, the USA's abilities to compound the pandemic actually stretch far beyond the powers of its pharmaceutical industrial complex.

As David Harvey notes, the creation of 'structural adjustment programs' has played a significant role in the movement of capital from the Global South to the Global North following the purging of Keynesian influences from the International Monetary Fund (IMF) and the World Bank. First implemented following the run on the dollar in 1980, such programs were designed to spread and consolidate neoliberal 'free market' orthodoxy by requiring indebted nations (primarily in Latin America and Africa) 'to implement institutional reforms, such as cuts in welfare expenditures, more flexible labour market laws, and privatization' in return for debt rescheduling (Harvey 2005, 29). While public healthcare services degraded, liberalized trade rules allowed investors to take over swathes of agricultural land in indebted countries, with devastating effects for employment rates.

Eswatini (also known as Swaziland – its former official name) represents an especially grave example of neoliberalism's global influence, as the country's 'once-thriving textile industry was flattened in 2005 when the WTO liberalized the global textile trade. Factories shut down overnight as producers relocated to Asia for cheaper labour, putting some 30,000 women instantly out of work' (Hickel 2013). Many such women turned to sex work as a means of survival, significantly catalyzing the spread of HIV/AIDS in Eswatini and surrounding areas. To add insult to injury, the US has continually obfuscated its role in prolonging the HIV/AIDS crisis through donations and charitable programs, such as the President's Emergency Program for AIDS Relief (PEPFAR). Introduced by President George W. Bush in 2003, PEPFAR is an HIV/AIDS prevention program targeting populations across 50 countries, primarily in Africa and Southeast Asia. Official government guidance characterizes PEPFAR as 'the largest commitment by any nation to address a single disease in history, enabled by strong bipartisan support across ten U.S. congresses and four presidential administrations, and through the American people's generosity', going on to explain how 'PEPFAR shows the power of what is possible through compassionate, cost-effective, accountable, and transparent American foreign assistance' (HIV.gov 2019). Underlying such rhetoric, however, are neocolonial endeavors to shore up consent for US hegemonic power.

When first introduced, a significant portion of PEPFAR's prevention strategies involved the provision of moralistic sex education promoting abstinence, faithful marriages, and condom use for those deemed to be 'high risk'. Such an approach obscured how material inequalities and expropriative structural adjustment programs have affected the spread of HIV, casting individuals and their supposedly poor choices as primarily responsible for the scale of the pandemic. By implication, therefore, the program classified those in its target countries as lacking the willpower and moral fortitude of an essentially superior American constituency, justifying US dominance and the imposition of neoliberal values. As Anthony M. Petro notes, this attitude represents a uniquely American form of religious power that is 'perhaps most visible in cases where it has been translated into a conventionally secular vocabulary, in both the moral language of health and medicine and in rhetoric about American citizenship and its limits' (Petro 2015, 4). As we will address in later chapters, neoconservative and far-right evangelicalism played a fundamental role in shaping the emergence of neoliberal hegemony in the late twentieth century, a legacy which continues to affect queer politics and HIV prevention today.

Substantiating (indeed, promoting) PEPFAR's role as a bulwark of US hegemony, Bush appointed Randall Tobias – the former head of major pharmaceutical company Eli Lilly – to head up the program. As Elisabeth Pisani and others have argued, the launch of PEPFAR served Tobias's class interests insofar as it guaranteed 'an extra two million patients for US drug manufacturers' amid dwindling market prospects (Pisani 2008, 215). As pharmaceutical companies in Global South countries like Brazil and India sold generic HIV/AIDS drugs at a fraction of the costs initially set by US Big Pharma, prices fell across the board. Initially stipulating that funds were to be channeled to US drug companies on the basis of safety and quality concerns, PEPFAR propped up an increasingly unprofitable industry segment in the early 2000s – just one example of the fallacy of 'free' markets under a neoliberal hegemony rigged in favor of the already powerful.

Although PEPFAR has liberalized its approach to generics and its strong opposition to practices like sex work over the years, it continues to assert US geopolitical dominance through something it terms 'blood security'. Blood security policies claim to protect the US citizenry from harm through rigorous collection and testing processes that promote the 'rational' use of blood 'products'. As Cathy Hannabach explains, PEPFAR's

> commodity-focused discourse of "quality assurance" and "rational use" reflects a neoliberal biopolitics that links blood to sex and race via security. This policy reflects intense racial, sexual, gender, and national violences as "bad blood" and "bad sex" are mapped onto racialized bodies in the global South that are positioned as security threats to the US and contemporary geopolitics. PEPFAR then seeks to manage the circulation of "bad blood/sex" in the name of protecting US political and economic interests. (Hannabach 2016, 117)

While US governance in the twenty-first century might have at least partially expunged the rabid homophobia and explicit racism seen in earlier discourses surrounding HIV/AIDS, its commitment to maintaining global hegemonic dominance through neoliberal 'free market' policies compounds historical inequalities – obstructing the action needed to effectively tackle the pandemic.

To summarize this abridged history, then, evidence of capitalism's insidious ability to exacerbate the HIV/AIDS pandemic abounds. Perhaps Schulman best sums up the impossible decisions facing groups like ACT UP, whose 'advocates were able, in a sense, to beat HIV', but 'could not beat capitalism' (Schulman 2021a, 10). The profit imperatives that drive and empower pharmaceutical companies preclude the equitable distribution of HIV medications to those who need them in the United States and beyond. As a result, 'around three-quarters of a million people throughout the world still die every year of a disease that is entirely manageable' (Schulman 2021a, 10). Despite such high levels of mortality, a person living in the Global North might be forgiven for believing the HIV/AIDS pandemic to be virtually over, or at least under control. Today, mainstream discourse surrounding the crisis tends to be concentrated around fictional or hagiographical portrayals of suffering among queer communities in affluent regions during the 1980s and how they eventually triumph in their efforts to secure life-saving treatment. At the same time, the continued effects of the virus on poorer countries and communities remain somewhat of an afterthought.

As Jih-Fei Cheng notes of David France's acclaimed documentary film, *How to Survive a Plague* (2012), which attempts to chronicle the history of the American epidemic, the director

> tells an incomplete, even false, story meant to convince audiences that biomedical interventions generated and distributed by corporate pharmaceuticals, like preexposure prophylaxis (PrEP), will solve the pandemic. However, this narrative of biomedical progress comes at the cost of jettisoning analysis about how the AIDS pandemic is historically and continually formed through structural inequalities experienced by nonwhite peoples who are denied biomedical access. (Cheng 2020, 81)

This story has been allowed to emerge in part due to the changing nature of neoliberal hegemony over the past couple of decades. The moralistic, socially conservative version of neoliberalism that emerged in the Thatcher and Reagan years was unsustainably coercive and self-contradictory, selling market freedoms while still 'somehow restrict[ing] the free movement of people', claiming to 'liberate the individual entrepreneur but somehow protect the nuclear family (Gilbert and Williams 2022, 4). The valorization of traditional gender roles is simply less tenable in a society where dwindling welfare provisions and an increasingly deregulated labor market leave many households unable to survive on a single wage.

What remained of neoliberal orthodoxy in the twenty-first century was, therefore, a commitment to trade liberalization and the empowerment of finance capital. The dominant hegemon's complicity in the HIV/AIDS crisis became less noticeable, seemingly outsourced to the whims of the market. Drained of their more extreme and quasi-fascistic approaches to the pandemic, the US and its neighbors in the Global North appeared to lead the world out of the darkest days of the crisis, buoyed by new charitable commitments to tackling HIV. As we will see, this teleology represents a tricky narrative with which to contend. While HIV/AIDS playwrights operating in the early years of the crisis could straightforwardly pinpoint the subjects of their ire (namely, Republican politicians in the US), increasing acceptance of queer relationships in the 1990s and early twenty-first century rendered the forces behind the continued spread of HIV increasingly abstract. This study, therefore, will untangle the ways in which playwrights addressing the HIV/AIDS crisis have grappled with the insidiously disempowering aspects of capitalism's latest, highly financialized phase.

Gramscian approaches to capitalist critique

Having established at least some of the ways in which capitalism and its neoliberal imperatives have hampered society's potential to tackle HIV/AIDS, I turn to the theoretical scholarship that underpins my critique of HIV/AIDS theater and its politics. In some ways, the 2020s represent a propitious vantage point from which to critique capitalism's neoliberal phase, ravaged as it is by hegemonic crises and existential threats. As Nancy Fraser puts it,

> Capitalism is back! After decades in which the term could scarcely be found outside the writings of Marxist thinkers, commentators of varying stripes now worry openly about its sustainability, scholars from every school scramble to systematize criticisms of it, and activists throughout the world mobilize in opposition to its practices. (Fraser 2022, 1)

As wealth inequality, climate breakdown, democratic crises, and social unrest intensify, capitalism's capacity to support a functional society or, indeed, a livable planet appears increasingly dubious. It should come as no surprise, therefore, that growing numbers of scholars and activists are returning to anti-capitalist ideas widely considered abandoned or debunked during the 1990s and 2000s – and, in turn, providing fresh theoretical frameworks through which to evaluate the socio-economic effects of decades' worth of neoliberal orthodoxy. Much anti-capitalist critique – while positioning itself within a wide array of political traditions and schools of thought – relies at least in part on Marxist theory, building on Marx's enduring insight that the personal relationships, roles, and institutions which make up the social fabric of capitalist society are shaped by a process known as alienation.

In simple terms, alienation occurs when a person's actions are subordinated to the needs of capital in ways that appears seamless and natural, while draining them of their humanity or 'species-being'; reducing workers to their ability to labor. The networks of human doing that help meet society's material needs are obfuscated by a mode of exchange in which the generation of profit and the accumulation of capital has become the driving force, such that

> the relations connecting the labour of one individual with that of the rest appear, not as social relations between individuals at work, but as what they really are, material relations between persons and social relations between things. It is only by being exchanged that the products of labour acquire, as values, one uniform social status, distinct from their varied forms of existence as objects of utility. (Marx 2013, 48)

In other words, capitalist systems are not interested in organizing the production of material goods around the fulfillment of human needs; rather, they rely on a competitive dynamism in which such needs are merely enmeshed. While useful labor (e.g., that which provides sustenance or shelter) continues to exist, the dynamics of capitalist exchange impose 'an abstraction which rebounds upon the way in which the concrete labour is performed' (Holloway 2010, 92).

The factory personnel working to produce drugs for pharmaceutical conglomerates, for example, are distanced from the effects their work has on the bodies of sick patients. Abstracted from the effects of this labor, their actions are motivated by the need to generate income and purchase necessities created by the hands of other alienated workers. This invisible connectedness of workers' actions is what makes capitalism so durable and seemingly impossible to undermine. What's more, the weaving together of invisible bonds 'is achieved not through the state (as appears to be the case) but through the abstraction of labour (the state is no more than a sort of protective coating that gives extra cement to the weave of abstraction)' (Holloway 2010, 95). Thus, capitalism weaves particular kinds of alienated doing into a totality that appears natural and unbreakable even to those politicians with the ostensible power to change things, thereby sanitizing and neutralizing the adverse events capitalism produces or catalyzes – such as the HIV/AIDS pandemic.

Of course, subsumption into such a totalizing and alienating system does not necessarily preclude dissent, critique, or subversion – as amply demonstrated by global histories of anti-capitalist organizing. As such, when capitalism's failures and injustices poke through the cracks of its foundations, those who bear the brunt of such systemic cruelties are incentivized to protect their material interests through a combination of actions such as protest, artistic production and expression, direct action, withdrawal of labor, organized violence, property destruction, rioting, and more. In response, dominant powers must find new tactics to maintain legitimacy within the social structures upon which they rely to generate wealth and material goods.

For the most part, anti-capitalist and social justice movements in the neoliberal states of the late twentieth and early twenty-first centuries have remained peaceful, comprising protest, art, and direct action. While many have garnered public attention, few have claimed tangible victories. ACT UP is an outlier in having successfully secured some of its demands, helping it become, as Schulman puts it, 'one of the most successful social movements in recent history' (Schulman 2021b). At the same time, the artistic products critiquing states' reactions to the HIV/AIDS crisis – such as Larry Kramer's *The Normal Heart* and Tony Kushner's *Angels in America* – remain a source of fascination for contemporary audiences who flock to revivals of early plays. Clearly, the art, protest, and direct actions of certain marginalized groups in the 1980s and 1990s played a crucial role in altering public perceptions of people living with HIV/AIDS.

To say such resistance significantly altered or undermined the wider neoliberal social relations that facilitated the initial spread of the virus, however, would be syllogistic. The links between the rise of neoliberalism and the failure to address HIV remain obfuscated outside of academic discourse – as demonstrated by the reception of popular cultural products such as the recent revival of *Angels* at London's National Theatre in 2017, directed by Marianne Elliott. For many, this much-anticipated run represented a sobering yet triumphal reminder of the extent to which contemporary liberal democracy has improved the lives of people with HIV/AIDS and queer communities since the dark days of the 1980s. A *Guardian* reviewer, for example, mused that 'Prejudice and homophobia still exist but, watching the first play, one is reminded how much has changed since it was written in terms of gay rights, sexual openness and HIV-testing' (Billington 2017), while a reviewer for *The Stage* explained that 'Where once it might have been a radical statement, *Angels in America* now plays like a raw, truthful documentary of where we've come from, and serves as a necessary reminder of those bleak times before AIDS became a treatable disease' (Shenton 2017). To historicize the HIV/AIDS crisis in such a way – ignoring the ways in which it continues to affect marginalized constituencies the world over – both writers must, to some extent, be inured to capitalism's iterative injustices and alienating functions. While the HIV pandemic has often worried at the fabric of neoliberalism's competitive and market-driven rationality, the nexus of corporations, state actors, wealthy individuals, and parties otherwise invested in neoliberalism's survival continue to maintain power and legitimacy.

With this in mind, the succeeding chapters will assess the extent to which HIV/AIDS theater and performance projects have threatened (or, indeed, upheld) the integrity of this alienating order. Some of the most effective theoretical tools with which to untangle this knotty line of enquiry reside in the works of Antonio Gramsci and the broader field of Gramscian cultural studies. From the cultural materialism of Raymond Williams to more recent post-Marxist critical theory, the ideas in which I am interested are primarily concerned with the role of hegemony – a constellation of various forms of power which seek to shape the beliefs, perceptions, and values of a given society (its 'common sense') – in preserving the dominance of a given social structure. As Stuart Hall explains, hegemonic authority extends far beyond the confines of electoral or party politics, constructed as it is 'in relation to political, moral, intellectual, cultural, ideological, sexual questions. The question of hegemony is always the question of a new cultural order' (Hall 2017). In other words, a significant component of hegemonic power lies in culture – a slippery, complex term that, for the purposes of this introduction, we will limit to those artistic products (plays, films, novels, performance art) that represent my objects of focus.

While Gramscian analysis builds on insights drawn from the work of Karl Marx and the Marxist tradition, its view of the cultural and economic as inextricable precipitated forms of analysis that diverged from Marxism's more orthodox articulations, casting a skeptical eye over arguments that supported, for example, the widely cited base–superstructure model. This idea separates the relations of production (the base) into a separate sphere from society's cultural forms, political ideas, and institutions (the superstructure), positing that the base primarily influences the formation of the superstructure. It has been heavily critiqued as a flawed metaphor that fails to account for the complex imbrications of such forces and for encouraging reductive interpretations of the ways in which ideologies, norms, and cultural assumptions are crystallized under capitalism. Cultural materialism represents one theoretical strand to have addressed this problem through examination of the relation between cultural production and the development of social relations in a given historical moment. Through revaluations of concepts such as the base, which came to be interpreted not as a fixed economic abstraction but as a description of shifting dynamic processes involving both social and economic activity, Raymond Williams claimed to arrive at cultural materialism as 'a theory of culture as a (social and material) productive process and of specific practices, of "arts", as social uses of material means of production (from language as material "practical consciousness" to the specific technologies of writing and forms of writing, through to mechanical and electronic communications systems)' (Williams 2005, 243). In this way, he was keen to emphasize the contribution of culture (broadly conceived) to the productive processes that shape society and, by extension, maintain or challenge dominant value systems and manifestations of power. Cultural products such as plays and novels (to pick forms with which Williams often engaged) do not merely represent the secondary effects of determining productive forces, but are themselves active elements in the construction of social realities.

Such an approach helps us avoid reducing the work of artists to products of either alienated labor or radically free expression and countercultural aspirations. As Michael Chanan notes, the artist has long been romanticized as operating outside of mainstream society's ideological imperatives – possessing intellectual autonomy 'bound up with a concept of individualism which has been paradigmatic for modern thought since the Enlightenment, if not the Renaissance, and only intensified by the Romantic turn to subjectivity and inner life' (Chanan 2022, 10). Cultural materialism asks us to disavow this enduring cultural narrative not through brute materialist abstraction but, rather, a view of cultural production and consumption as reciprocal. The impetus behind labor cannot be reduced to the need to generate means for survival (although this need often plays a significant role). Different kinds of labor – to varying extents – also contain cultural dimensions, allowing workers to freely mobilize their imaginations and physical skills to engage in purposeful activities. Under the capitalist mode of production, however, work is significantly drained of its self-fulfilling qualities, propelled by the promises of wages rather than inventive or artistic motivations. Despite this structural antagonism to satisfactory labor, creativity 'persists, in various forms of labour where the worker retains an element of control over the labour process over which the capitalist is unable to impose regulation, or can only do so imperfectly' (Chanan 2022, 16). Negotiating this space between artistic production as self-fulfillment and artistic production as bound to the exigencies of capitalist accumulation is especially vital – and challenging – within our current neoliberal conjuncture.

On one hand, the last several decades have witnessed an ever-intensifying cultural emphasis on the value of competition, individualism, and self-sufficiency as justification for the kind of neoliberal deregulatory economic frameworks that strip workers of job security, bargaining power, and protection from exploitative practices. As well as impacting how capital flows through the international monetary system and inaugurating a new era of finance capital and market deregulation, neoliberal philosophies etch themselves on our malleable subjectivities, affecting our everyday decisions and interactions. Consequently, artistic talent is frequently conceptualized as a kind of useful asset, the primary benefit of which is enhanced employability within a competitive jobs market. Shackled by the need to reproduce themselves through wage labor, the proletarianized artist is compelled to apply their talents to projects that uphold the status quo upon which their income relies. As Delgado and Svich's volume attests, this neoliberal landscape has helped digestible, normative, unchallenging theater proliferate.

On the other hand, this line of argument risks indulging in a kind of rhetorical overcorrection. Take, for example, John Holloway's description of capitalism's alienating function in his polemical *Crack Capitalism* (2010). To illustrate the ways in which capitalism drains one of autonomy in one's labor, he takes the example of a cake-making hobbyist who decides to make their love of baking into a full-time job. Once the cake-making process is weighed down by the need to make a profit, he explains, it loses its enjoyable aspects:

> After a while I realise that I am not earning enough money and think that, since cake-making is in any case merely a means to an end, a way of earning money, I might as well make something else that will sell better. My doing has become completely indifferent to its content, there has been a complete abstraction from its concrete characteristics. The object I produce is now so completely alienated from me that I do not care whether it is a cake or rat poison, as long as it sells. (Holloway 2010, 93)

While the scenario Holloway describes here is helpfully illustrative of capitalism's alienating function and vicious imperatives, such a trajectory is by no means inevitable. To say capitalism is capable of *completely* detaching one's doing from its concrete characteristics is, perhaps, to overstate or simplify the power of the profit motive. A cake maker, for example, might happily compromise the quality of their ingredients to improve return on investment while retaining some pleasure and pride in producing cakes that bring joy to clients. While they might not be able to extricate themselves from the demands of the market, they might be able to navigate its demands in such a way as to retain a kernel of what Holloway terms 'conscious doing' – actions that retain prosocial or self-fulfilling motives. Similarly, a theater maker or dramaturg might carefully negotiate the demands of profit-seeking arts institutions unwilling to stage or promote 'risky' work that might not appeal to audiences or might threaten a theater's reputation. While they might not enjoy creative sovereignty, they might push institutional boundaries or experiment with novel ways to circumnavigate normative strictures and tell new stories about topics such as HIV/AIDS. Capitalism's regulatory function might be powerful, but, as Chanan notes, it is less than perfect when we consider forms of labor requiring creative skills and imaginative capacities.

So, how can we parse the extent to which individual plays capitulate to the demands of the neoliberal theater? And, indeed, the extent to which playwrights might critique capitalism's role in worsening the HIV/AIDS crisis from within such an institution? As we will see throughout the coming chapters, this task demands that we view neoliberalism's common-sense narratives as always fragile, fragmentary, and vulnerable to critique. Common sense, according to Gramsci, reflects

> the conception of the world which is uncritically absorbed by the various social and cultural environments in which the moral individuality of the average man is developed. Common sense is not a single unique conception, identical in time and space. It is the "folklore" of philosophy, and, like folklore, it takes countless different forms. Its most fundamental characteristic is that it is a conception which, even in the brain of one individual, is fragmentary, incoherent and inconsequential, in conformity with the social and cultural position of those masses whose philosophy it is. (Gramsci 2003, 419)

Common-sense ideas, then, are those that are easily digested and absorbed by dint of their seemingly indubitable nature. They reflect the commonly held beliefs of a given moment and comprise seemingly obvious ideas that shape its moral fabric. Common sense is, in essence, 'a compendium of well-tried knowledge, customary beliefs, wise sayings, popular nostrums and prejudices, some of which – like "a little of what you fancy does you good" – seem eminently sensible, others wildly inaccurate' (Hall and O'Shea 2013, 9). Gramsci's notion of common sense therefore provides an explicatory framework through which to understand how dominant powers inculcate citizens – including marginalized people, activists, and artists – into a worldview that valorizes individualism and free-market fundamentalism. At the same time, its fragmentary and contingent nature offers opportunities to reveal how contemporary social relations and material interests uphold such a worldview – and, therefore, its failures and injustices.

From a Gramscian perspective, then, neoliberalism is a complex and often contradictory aggregation of common-sense ideas and beliefs that conspire to tell the neoliberal agent that she is 'all at once the business, the raw material, the product, the clientele, and the customer of her own life. She is a jumble of assets to be invested, nurtured, managed and developed' (Mirowski 2014, 108). Even institutions and political actors with contradictory values work to achieve this 'all-at-once'-ness if it suits their material interests, covering up any ideological contradictions with seemingly innocuous and obvious axioms. The neoliberal agent might believe that her consumer power, for example, offers a fabulous degree of personal freedom. However, the power to exercise such freedom is often dependent on the successful navigation of an increasingly corporate labor market that demands the fulfillment of evermore stringent (and decidedly subjugating) personal targets and performance appraisals.

Common-sense neoliberalism does not work so covertly as to be invisible, however. It is a named phenomenon enthusiastically derided by throngs of scholars and political commentators, after all, demonstrating a healthy degree of conscious opposition to its effects. Such opposition typically appears as what Williams describes as 'emergent' phenomena. In contradistinction to residual culture – elements of which, despite being formed in the relatively distant past, are still often active in the cultural process – the emergent involves the creation of 'new meanings and values, new practices, new relationships and kinds of relationship' that do not merely represent 'some new phase of the dominant culture' (Williams 1989, 123). Emergent culture must, strictly speaking, offer alternative or oppositional modes of thought and expression because, 'since we are always considering relations within a cultural process, definitions of the emergent, as of the residual, can be made only in relation to a full sense of the dominant' or hegemonic (Williams 1989, 123). Emergent movements, in other words, steer hegemony's shape-shifting quality, altering society's class composition, recalibrating widespread common-sense notions, and, in some cases, altering themselves to fit into existing hegemonic forms. As Hall so concisely puts it, 'No project achieves "hegemony" as a completed project. It is a process, not a state of being. No victories are permanent or final. Hegemony has constantly to be "worked on", maintained, renewed, revised' (Hall 2011, 26). When hegemonic ideas fail to achieve the consent of certain social groups, resistance movements or counterhegemonic strategies bubble up. Over time, significant resistance to contemporary paradigms might create a hegemonic crisis, in which countervailing forces might tussle for dominance.

This book will track this constant negotiation between consent and opposition within HIV/AIDS theater, assessing the extent to which the genre is capable of spreading and legitimizing emergent ideas. I start by analyzing early plays with which readers are most likely to be familiar, assessing the legacy of what are commonly referred to as 'AIDS plays' in scholarly literature and wider culture by discussing the politics of revision, reexamination, and revival in neoliberal times. Next, I assess some of the twentieth century's lesser-known AIDS plays, situating their production within a wider context of burgeoning neoliberal politics and examining their creators' willingness to stage 'queerer' dramaturgies in contradistinction to their more widely acclaimed peers. I then move to examine HIV/AIDS theater in the twenty-first century, assessing the political dimensions of its cleavage into loose sub-categories (some of which overlap) – public-health-oriented work, plays targeted at racialized and otherwise marginalized communities peripheral to white queer constituencies, subcultural (often solo) performance work that takes aim at capitalism's subjugating functions, and historically oriented work that tracks the development of HIV/AIDS and queer politics over time. In following the development of HIV/AIDS theater in this way, selecting some of the best-known or most illustrative exemplars from each thematic and periodized category, I engage in a form of conjunctural analysis. Grounded in the Gramscian tradition and developed by the likes of cultural studies scholars such as Stuart Hall, conjunctural analysis interprets cultural products as actively involved in generating the ideas and institutions that either extend the life of dominant political paradigms ('conjunctures') or participate in creating new ones. As Deborah Grayson and Ben Little explain, conjunctural analysis views crises that threaten the material wellbeing of the majority (such as climate change) as driving hegemonic change. It helps identify the 'potential for movement between one settlement and the next at times when the existing tendencies of a society [...] exhaust their possibilities for renewal, and a new organisation of social forces is required'

(Grayson and Little 2017, 63). Such an approach therefore necessitates the combination of close textual analysis with analysis of the wider political, economic, and cultural ecology within which performance works intervene, helping us assess how hegemonic shifts of the past four decades have satisfied the interests of audiences or, indeed, left them unfulfilled.

How does existing HIV/AIDS theater scholarship address capitalism?

In homing in on the genre's most widely disseminated, revived, and lauded plays, this book encroaches on well-trodden ground. While this approach might seem to recapitulate the exclusionary trappings of previous scholarship, its Gramscian underpinnings will, I hope, helpfully elucidate the material bases upon which well-known HIV/AIDS plays have built their popular appeal. The coincidental rise of neoliberalism in tandem with the emergence of the HIV/AIDS pandemic remains undertheorized in current theater scholarship, glossing over how capitalism's distributive and hegemonic functions have secured the supremacy of a few select plays in the HIV/AIDS theater canon. This is not to say that scholarship has completely overlooked the political economic dimensions of HIV/AIDS theater. David Román's *Acts of Intervention: Performance, Gay Culture, and AIDS* (1998), for example, which examines the ways in which gay men have used theater as a political tool, acknowledges how the

> economics of performance, like the economics of AIDS, conditions and disciplines bodies into a hegemonic norm that assumes neutrality and fixity. The political and ideological marks of these systems that produce AIDS and that produce theatre, if unchecked, remain veiled and thereby assume a privileged site of truth, of claims to the real. (Román 1998, 149)

Many of the early HIV/AIDS plays Román addresses – from the solo work of Ron Vawter and Tim Miller to Kushner's *Angels* – he claims agitate such hegemonic norms in a bid to alter popular, often stigmatizing narratives about AIDS and queer communities.

Beyond this study, Kushner's work has inspired much debate on how it employs historical materialist ideas, with scholars such as David Savran questioning whether *Angels'* Marxist allusions carry any substantive counterhegemonic potential. Savran acknowledges

Kushner's avowed commitment to socialism and intellectual critique of hegemony in late twentieth-century America. However, he also harbors suspicions that 'as a member of the bourgeoisie and as the recipient of two Tony awards, [Kushner] is also committed – if only unconsciously – to the continuation of the system that has granted him no small measure of success' (Savran 1995, 226). While such critique pinpoints capitalism's antagonistic role in the production of HIV/AIDS theater, it ignores the fact that few playwrights have paid as much attention as Kushner to this question of political economy since the 1990s – when neoliberalism was in an earlier hegemonic stage. As we will see, the twenty-first century has precipitated a rise in assimilatory HIV/AIDS theater willing to adopt normative modes of thinking that would have scandalized some of its more radical predecessors. Today, common-sense neoliberal notions surrounding healthcare and community care have interpenetrated the genre to such an extent that it has become less about pushing back against oppressive societal forces and more about celebrating progress in treatment regimens and disseminating public health information. As such, there has also been an unwillingness to read early HIV/AIDS plays alongside later works or, indeed, view HIV-related theater as containing common themes worthy of comparison and critique – something this book attempts to rectify.

In tandem with this strengthening of neoliberal hegemony, some twenty-first-century scholarship has skirted around critique of HIV/AIDS plays' entanglement with capitalist social relations, arguing that their affective power possesses liberatory potential. Jacob Juntunen's *Mainstream AIDS Theatre, the Media, and Gay Civil Rights: Making the Radical Palatable* (2016), for example, accuses scholars such as Román – who engages in some materialist analysis – of employing ideology in a 'particularly pessimistic Marxist fashion'. He claims that what he demarcates as 'mainstream' HIV/AIDS plays 'simultaneously incorporate elements of an emergent ideology while reproducing enough of the dominant ideology to be palatable within the culture industry', thus bolstering the acceptance of gay men within the 'U.S. imagined community' and alleviating some of the stigma surrounding HIV/AIDS (Juntunen 2016, 26). In other words, US audiences of mainstream theater are more likely to feel a strong affinity with, or sympathy for, 'middle-class, white, HIV-positive gay men' onstage compared to characters who fall outside of this constrictive group (Juntunen 2016, 19). Relatedly, he believes early AIDS plays such as *The Normal Heart* entered the cultural mainstream by making palatable aspects of 'gay culture' that lay too far outside the confines of respectable 'straight culture'. While Juntunen acknowledges the dangers of establishing 'a marriage/promiscuity binary at the heart of AIDS', he ultimately argues in favor of this binary for its ability to make 'the play's messages easier for the dominant ideology to assimilate' (Juntunen 2016, 44). While Juntunen might be correct in his assertion that Kramer's anti-sex approach softened attitudes among straight liberals or those on the center-right, he does not explicitly address how such a gradualist approach would work when it comes to providing marginalized groups with the material support they require to weather a virus such as HIV – especially at a time when a staunchly right-wing, evangelical-aligned government was in office.

So, in consonance with neoliberalism's ostensible faith in the rational, autonomous individual as driver of societal progress, Juntunen conceptualizes stigma as epiphenomenal yet somehow mutable via gentle emotional persuasion. Although he deploys the language of cultural materialism in separating emergent from dominant ideologies, he largely sidesteps the economic and material dimensions of power, viewing social progression as operating almost entirely at the superstructural level. Representation, for Juntunen, is enough to drive change. Kalle Westerling, writing during the presidency of Donald Trump, notes that this line of argument betrays 'an incredibly hopeful, almost utopian sense of optimism and progress, written before the current US presidency. [Juntunen's] arguments about continual progress must overlook that the crisis of HIV/AIDS in both the United States and globally is still ongoing' (Westerling 2018, 128). While I do not doubt that assimilatory representation plays a role in softening public attitudes toward certain minority groups, I am unconvinced that such politically compromised forms of cultural production are necessarily steps on the road to social justice. Quite the contrary, this kind of cozy politics can obscure the ways in which exploitation occurs under neoliberal capitalism, while reassuring audiences that their newfound sympathies with those Juntunen terms 'victims' of AIDS are enough to remedy decades of marginalization.

Of course, given the increasing public consciousness surrounding intersecting forms of marginalization (at least for those of a more socially liberal persuasion), the politics of representation are moving away from the relative conservatism Juntunen describes. While mainstream cultural production about the HIV/AIDS crisis remains largely centered on the white, gay, male experience – Robin Campillo's film *120 BPM* (2017) or theatrical and on-screen revivals of older AIDS plays, for example – works such as the TV drama series *Pose* (2018–21) have garnered praise for breaking this representational mold. *Pose* chronicles the effects of HIV/AIDS on a group of close-knit individuals involved in New York's largely Black and Latinx underground ballroom culture, some of whom are transgender, sex workers, or both. In one sense, representing the experiences of queer people of color and, indeed, transgender sex workers of color who remain viciously monstered in contemporary culture can be seen as a corrective to the sanitized depictions of AIDS Juntunen favors. As *Variety* critic Caroline Framke puts it, *Pose* 'devotes the kind of attention (and budget) that typically goes to conflicted straight male antiheros to the glittering grunge of New York City's ballroom scene circa 1987' (Framke 2018). Thus, it centers the experiences of historically marginalized communities in a bid to push back against hegemonic prejudices. However, as Laura Stamm notes, the historical moment in which *Pose* takes place is distant enough to harbor depoliticizing effects, implying that 'trans women and the queer community no longer have something to protest' (Stamm 2020, 617).

Certainly, the affective dimensions of *Pose* should be read alongside the commercial exigencies of the contemporary television industry to comprehend how such depoliticization takes place. While the ballroom scene the show portrays might have operated on a countercultural plain in the 1980s and 1990s, the semiotics of vogueing and drag culture have somewhat altered in recent years thanks to their mainstreaming by the likes of hit reality television show *Ru Paul's Drag Race*. Framke, for example, expresses doubts as to the number of younger viewers who would know where their favorite *Drag Race* catchphrases came from without *Pose*. The latter educates them by platforming the 'queer and trans people of color whose ingenuity could make even the dingiest of spaces come alive', aiming 'to make that oft-buried history vibrant and current, with all the glitter and heft that FX can give it' (Framke 2018). Although such glamorization celebrates difference and individual expression in a way that challenges normative ideals surrounding gender and sexuality, the commercialization of drag and queer culture within the mainstream distracts us from the material inequities experienced by minoritized groups – a small price to pay, no doubt, for the television companies whose bottom line relies on pleasing their audiences and outcompeting an ever-growing collection of streaming services.

The glitz of *Pose* successfully satisfies hegemonic ideals by casting the 'dinginess' (read: dispossession) Framke describes as an obstacle for the show's protagonists to fight and overcome through their essential ingenuity. Such a narrative is highly compatible with neoliberal ideals of self-sufficiency and competition, ignoring the ways in which the material dispossession of minoritized groups systematically renders them vulnerable to health issues such as HIV/AIDS. Such a cozily hegemonic historicization of transgender experiences of HIV/AIDS fails to contextualize an ongoing crisis in which 'transfeminine people of colour face extremely high rates of HIV infection due to poverty, sex work, and exposure to violence. According to several urban needs assessment surveys in major US cities, HIV infection among trans women of colour exceeded 80%' (O'Brien 2021, 56). While tales of individual overcoming and the celebration of difference might satisfy audiences and affirm hegemonic understandings of the world, they do not raise consciousness about the extent and urgency of the HIV pandemic.

Thanks to the popularity of digestible cultural products such as *Pose*, it remains the case that stories of the contemporary effects of HIV/AIDS on marginalized constituencies rarely enter mainstream cultural discourse. This is not to say, of course, that theater addressing the experiences of the global majority does not exist. To the contrary, underground, amateur, and shoestring theater and performance art has always operated as a counterhegemonic force within the wider politics of HIV/AIDS – exegeses of which have appeared in various academic volumes and sometimes even popular histories of the pandemic. Robb Hernandez's *Archiving an Epidemic: Art, AIDS, and the Queer Chicanx Avant-Garde* (2019), for example, conducts what the author terms 'queer detrital analyses' of both visual and performance art – a form of historiography that 'makes AIDS losses tangible through physical substitutions and reproductions of nonextant works' (Hernandez 2019, 23). In collating the remaining scraps of artists' oeuvres, assessing artists' involvement in commercial media, and listening to the experiences of marginal voices who witnessed the Chicanx art scene, Hernandez recovers histories typically drowned out by those of artists with greater cultural power.

Alyson Campbell and Dirk Gindt's edited volume of essays, *Viral Dramaturgies: HIV and AIDS in Performance in the Twenty-First Century* (2018), meanwhile, addresses HIV/AIDS performance work across a wide range of localities, including South Africa, Papua New Guinea, Sweden, Puerto Rico, China, and Canada. In so doing, its authors explore how contemporary theater makers and performers are worrying at the boundaries of a homogeneous HIV/AIDS theater genre – what Campbell and Gindt claim is 'still a burgeoning, ever-shifting field' inviting study 'of the manifold ways in which performance reflects and addresses the social and political challenges presently posed by HIV and AIDS' (Campbell and Gindt 2018, 5–6). Another body of work explores how community and applied forms of theater are working to prevent the ongoing spread of the virus, much of which focuses on theater producers in Africa. Examples include Ola Johansson's *Community Theatre and AIDS* (2011) and Hazel Barnes' *Applied Drama and Theatre as an Interdisciplinary Field in the Context of HIV/AIDS in Africa* (2014), both of which address forms of theater far removed from celebrity-filled productions of *Angels in America* to focus on the role of theater in sex and HIV awareness education.

While each of these volumes goes some way to plugging representational lacunae in HIV/AIDS theater scholarship or, indeed, directly examining how their case studies interact with neoliberal capitalism, the genre's development in co-incidence with late twentieth- and early twenty-first-century neoliberalism remains untheorized. In addressing this problem, this book accounts for the ways in which neoliberalism – which has shaped the uneven trajectory of the HIV/AIDS pandemic – has also shaped cultural consumption and public consciousness surrounding the virus. Given the enduring weight of theatrical work within the wider nexus of cultural production surrounding HIV/AIDS, a materialist reading will offer insights into why and how certain narratives about the virus remain.

Such a line of enquiry will have implications for scholarship beyond the realms of theater. Much cultural production surrounding HIV/AIDS – including some of the decade's most highly acclaimed television shows – appears to have adopted a kind of nostalgic tenor that erroneously casts the pandemic as over. As Stamm notes of *Pose*, 'the show has aired contemporaneously with other series that place HIV/AIDS in the 1980s past, including Netflix's *Glow* and HBO's *Deuce*', revealing a generalized nostalgia for the period, as well as a nostalgia for AIDS (Stamm 2020, 621). While the recent revivification of HIV/AIDS narratives represents a positive opportunity to destigmatize positive diagnoses and raise awareness about inequities surrounding drug provision, many widely praised cultural products fall well short of this mark. Russell T. Davies's recent transatlantic televisual hit *It's a Sin* (2021), for example, engages in a distinctly neoliberal and non-solidaristic kind of historiography in its depiction of stigma and homophobia in 1980s Britain. As Brian Mullin notes, 'structures of blame and mysteries of transmission drive the narrative', as Ritchie, the protagonist of the series, continues to have unprotected sex with scores of men following a positive diagnosis. Blaming such behavior on Ritchie's repressed and homophobic family unit, Davies 'paints a portrait of young men so crippled by homophobia that they lack any responsibility or ethics and pursue sex as a symptom of shame' and ensures the series 'elicits pity rather than solidarity' (Mullin 2021).

In casting its minoritized characters as subjects to be pitied, *It's a Sin* indulges viewers looking for sentimental storylines and reassurances about their empathetic capacities, while pathologizing queer communities for transgressing diktats surrounding personal responsibility. This volume provides urgent ways to critique such sentimentalism, seductive as it is. As we will see, understanding how contemporary political structures perpetuate the HIV pandemic requires an assiduous willingness to criticize even some of the most rhetorically appealing and seemingly righteous cultural products.

A summary of upcoming chapters

I begin my investigation by tracking the ways in which sentimental and pathologizing narratives surrounding HIV/AIDS have gained such adulation on the contemporary stage and in wider popular culture. Indeed, Chapter 1 refines existing critiques of so-called 'AIDS nostalgia' – a tendency to romanticize the pandemic and confine it to the past – through the lens of political economy. Starting with Larry Kramer's *The Normal Heart* and Swedish television series *Torka aldrig tårar utan handskar* [*Don't Ever Wipe Tears Without Gloves*] (based on Jonas Gardell's *Ömheten* [*Tenderness*]), I consider how the neoliberalization of theater as an institution incentivizes the continued production of plays promoting assimilatory sexual practices via narratively traditional love stories, as well as the ways in which sentimentality blinds spectators to the pandemic's cruel endurance. While normative storylines might have played a vital political function in softening attitudes toward queer constituencies during the early years of the crisis, their continued dominance in cultural production surrounding HIV/AIDS precludes our capacity to move toward a more solidaristic politics that adequately confronts the politico-economic structures perpetuating the negative impacts of HIV on marginalized constituencies. With this in mind, I move on to examine Tony Kushner's much-discussed *Angels in America*, examining its resistance to nostalgic impulses and commitment to a quasi-Brechtian dialectics that lays the groundwork for renewed counterhegemonic thinking – even three decades after its premiere. While acknowledging the play's many lacunae and limitations – especially regarding the imbrications of class, race and, gender-based inequities – I reestablish the play's socialistic potential amid growing scholarly criticism and demonstrate that AIDS nostalgia is by no means an inevitability or an intrinsic aspect of early HIV/AIDS plays.

Having reevaluated some of the HIV/AIDS genre's best-known plays, I turn my attention to a cohort of lesser-known playwrights willing to experiment with form and push back against the hegemonic order. Chapter 2 digs down into so-called 'second-generation' HIV/AIDS theater – a largely American subgenre that embraced 'queerer' dramaturgies in a bid to undermine homophobic and stigmatizing rhetoric perpetuated by high-profile institutions and political figures in the 1980s and 1990s. Second-generation plays went some way toward challenging assimilatory narratives and raising consciousness about late twentieth-century capitalism's role in subjugating gay men, particularly in the first years of the pandemic. I take Paul Rudnick's *The Most Fabulous Story Ever Told* – a queer reimagining of the story of Genesis – and solo performer Tim Miller's *My Queer Body* to examine the second generation's ability to identify and undermine strategic coalitions between neoliberal and neoconservative swathes of America's right wing. While understanding such plays today requires a nuanced appreciation of their historical context, their subsumption into America's late twentieth-century culture wars offers broader insights into neoliberal hegemonic tactics. Although religious and traditionally conservative groups might undermine the libertarianism of many neoliberal ideologues, their ability to whip up culture wars plays a useful role in distracting from the failures of the so-called free market.

I ultimately contend that many second-generation plays overlooked the inadequacy of capitalism to fight the pandemic *tout court*, especially in their inability to look beyond the queer community alone as an agent for positive change. In appealing and speaking to a largely homogeneous, metropolitan audience, they ignore the neglect of racialized people disproportionately affected by HIV/AIDS and adopt a politics with shallow horizons surrounding care, solidarity, and sexuality. An exception I identify toward the latter part of this chapter is Iranian-American playwright Reza Abdoh, whose experimental, sensorial, and often shocking dramaturgy confronts liberal audiences with their own complicity in the capitalist structures that perpetuate suffering among marginalized groups, including racialized people and people with HIV/AIDS. Spurred on by the fact of his own AIDS diagnosis and the attendant socio-economic structures aiding his corporeal decline, Abdoh's work is easily some of the most pointedly anti-capitalist featured in this book. Given the relatively lack of scholarly attention paid to his plays, I hope my analysis of such plays as *Bogeyman* and *The Law of*

Remains goes some way to re-popularizing Abdoh as an HIV/AIDS playwright, while demonstrates just some of the potentialities of the stage as a political tool in any anti-capitalist project.

Chapter 3 continues my examination of Reza Abdoh's body of work, focusing on the racial politics of the HIV/AIDS theater canon and assessing the absence of plays examining the effects of the virus on communities of color. While Abdoh stands out as a second-generation playwright willing to confront racial disparities, his provocative tactics might not reflect the kinds of solidaristic politics necessary to address the scale of the HIV/AIDS pandemic – a problem I examine closely in the first section of this chapter. Next, I turn my attention to the Pomo Afro Homos – a Black theater group operating around the same time as Abdoh and other second-generation playwrights. As well as critiquing the oversights of a largely white theater landscape, the Pomos examined prejudices within America's Black communities, contributing a much-needed political economy of stigma to HIV/AIDS theater. Acutely aware of the class interests behind America's culture wars, the Pomos represent a vital – albeit short-lived – juncture in the history of Black, gay representation within the genre.

The second half of Chapter 3 moves on to explore the paucity of Black radical HIV/AIDS theater following the Pomos' disbanding. While acknowledging that the absence of racialized constituencies onstage is substantially overdetermined, I argue that capitalism's alienating and expropriative functions play a significant role in curtailing certain forms of representation within the genre. As well as examining the whitewashing of HIV/AIDS theater via materialist critique, I analyze some of the genre's few commercial plays to address Black subjectivities and experiences of the virus, including Sarah Hall's immersive play *As Much as I Can*. I identify some of the ways in which contemporary Black HIV/AIDS plays address disproportionate infection rates through neoliberal solutions, adopting a form of art-cum-public-health measure that individualizes transmission risk and ultimately serves hegemonic ends. In so doing, I emphasize the difficulty of staging counterhegemonic plays in a way that adequately accounts for the imbrication of class, race, and identity issues under neoliberalism.

Finally, this chapter attends to one of the more confrontational and experimental Black HIV/AIDS plays to have recently emerged in the US – Donja R. Love's *one in two*. Love's play reflects on the inadequacy of the contemporary theater as a space for generative political reflection and solidarity, inhabited as it so often is by elite constituencies whose gaze might fetishize or otherize the Black body onstage. While *one in two* slickly critiques the socio-economic foundations of disparities in provision of HIV/AIDS care, my analysis struggles to find a generative way forward within this critique, posing questions about the future study and development of HIV/AIDS theater.

Chapter 4 extends my critique of public-health-oriented plays, examining a range of theatrical attempts to educate audiences about HIV/AIDS in the twenty-first century. Such plays appear to offer clear, politically neutral, and comprehensive information about the virus, albeit in an often sanitized and artless fashion. Underlying their core messages, however, are distinctly neoliberal public health imperatives designed to reduce HIV transmission by individualizing responsibility and pathologizing those who engage in subcultural forms of queer sex and sociality. I use a range of recent plays as case studies to reveal how pathologizing narratives often undergird a supposed ethos of anti-prejudice, starting with Peter Darney's *Five Guys Chillin'*, an example of documentary theater. Based partly or entirely on the testimony of real-life subjects, documentary theater comprises a substantial trend within the HIV/AIDS genre, harnessing the supposed verity of its storylines to garner audience sympathy and open their eyes to the realities of HIV/AIDS in the twenty-first century. Darney's play focuses on the subcultural practice of chemsex, attempting to humanize its participants in the face of moral panic whipped up by mainstream media. As I explain via critique of neoliberal therapy culture and individualized approaches to wellbeing, the play's inability to break away from hegemonic healthcare paradigms means it lacks the politics of interdependence and communality required to effectively rebuke stigmatizing notions. While *5 Guys Chillin'* offers some scope for educating audiences about the undeniable dangers of chemsex, its content and form fail to critique the structural and material foundations from which such dangers emerge, throwing up wider questions about the ethics and representational politics of documentary theater *tout court*.

Turning my attention to experimental dramaturgies much less interested in true-to-life stories, I analyze Lachlan Philpott's *Bison*, a play whose fragmented style mimics the immediacy and market-like structure of online hookup apps. In so doing, Philpott tells a story of solipsistic and destructive hedonism that compounds stigma surrounding HIV, while threatening to reverse progress made in containing the virus. I examine the political potentialities of this critique in the context of wider arguments surrounding online promiscuity and individual responsibility, ultimately arguing that the demands of medicalized discourses surrounding intimacy often curtail the ability of playwrights to think more expansively about the social and political functions of sex at a moment still rife with moralism and fear of the queer.

The final section of this chapter looks for work more willing to look beyond hegemonic health paradigms. In so doing, it briefly looks beyond the strictures of those mainstream cultural institutions more likely to receive funding from the government, private sector, or third sector, toward subcultural work emerging in more informal settings. Specifically, I examine moments from David Hoyle's *Magazine*, a series of performance-art-cum-stand-up shows that took place at London's Royal Vauxhall Tavern and addressed a range of hot social topics. While this choice of case study might seem to move beyond the confines of theater and into the realm of performance art or amateur comedy, the porous boundaries between these categories can tell us something about the politics of cultural production and HIV/AIDS. As my examination of Hoyle's work demonstrates, performances less beholden to theatrical norms might help elucidate some of the political constraints of the more mainstream work taking place under the proscenium arch. Such performances therefore provide hopeful insights into the potential for alternative pedagogical dramaturgies to emerge outside of a neoliberalized public health arena.

Acknowledging the difficulty of staging counterhegemonic plays given the shape of the contemporary economy, Chapter 5 considers how changing funding models within the arts over the past four decades have shaped the trajectory of HIV/AIDS theater. As well as examining the decimation of state-sponsored arts funding, I examine the phenomenon of crowdfunding and the increasing need for playwrights to bend to the whims of the so-called free market. As part of this analysis, I track the attempts of playwright Shaun Kitchener to crowdfund his play *Positive*, an awareness-raising play designed to reduce stigma surrounding HIV through a simple and educative storyline. While *Positive* represents an earnest attempt at improving public attitudes toward people with HIV, the promotional material used to promote the play reveals some of the creatively and politically inhibiting imperatives playwrights like Kitchener face when staging plays without traditional institutional funding. While the digital revolution and the rise of crowdfunding might appear to offer opportunities for dissident online communities to come together and create counterhegemonic work, this chapter critiques how the increased pressure to 'market' oneself and one's projects tends to quash such utopian dreaming. However, I end the chapter on a more hopeful note, identifying the relatively inexpensive nature of solo performance as a means for theater makers to galvanize their audiences on a shoestring budget. I examine Alexis Gregory's *Riot Act* – a pedagogical work examining the history of LGBTQ+ activism through the testimony of those involved in critical political events – and Neil Watkins' *The Year of Magical Wanking*, a crowdfunded autobiographical monologue that consciously rejects some of the compromises playwrights make when accepting donations, as well as the neoliberal ethics of self-care that undergirds many contemporary HIV/AIDS plays.

Finally, Chapter 6 takes stock of the state of HIV/AIDS theater at a time of hegemonic crisis. I look at the ways in which recent plays betray a commitment to what Nancy Fraser terms 'progressive neoliberalism' – an ideology that appears to advocate for the equal rights and economic freedoms of people across a broad range of constituencies through corporate 'diversity' rhetoric and appeals to meritocracy. While progressive neoliberalism is a formidable opponent for the more reactionary elements of the conservative right, it lacks the political consciousness necessary to combat capitalism's continued subjugation of queer, racialized, and gendered individuals. With this in mind, I assess how two major HIV/AIDS plays – *The Inheritance* by Matthew Lopez and *The Gay Heritage Project* by Damien Atkins, Paul Dunn, and Andrew Kushnir – address what 'progress' should look like in an age when the HIV pandemic and, indeed, a wider constellation of environmental and medical crises continues to wreak havoc on marginalized constituencies across the world. Both, I argue, offer formulations inadequate to the task of undermining capitalism's cruelties, limited as they are by a kind of romantic queer historicism. While some formulation of 'progress' is, of course, necessary in the fight against HIV/AIDS, the genre currently lacks a politics of interdependency capable of confronting the world's contemporary constellation of crises.

CHAPTER ONE

The Nostalgic Commodification of HIV/AIDS Theater

The medico-political fabric of the HIV/AIDS pandemic in the Global North has evolved considerably since the so-called 'crisis years', primarily due to the advancement of life-prolonging treatment regimens.[1] However, public knowledge surrounding the history of the crisis remains relatively impoverished, with many theatergoers craving enlightenment via digestible onstage narratives of suffering, death, and (often bittersweet) overcoming. As such, an increasing number of theater makers are producing revivals of HIV/AIDS plays originally performed in the 1980s and early 1990s for twenty-first-century audiences. Larry Kramer's polemic *The Normal Heart* (1985), for example, which follows a group of gay New Yorkers and activists grappling with the crisis in the early 1980s, has been restaged to transatlantic acclaim across several theaters, including Broadway's Golden Theatre in 2011, Toronto's Buddies in Bad Times Theatre in 2012, and London's National Theatre in 2021. William Hoffman's *As Is* (1985), meanwhile, which deals with similar themes to Kramer's play, has graced a variety

1 I deploy the term 'crisis years' in scare quotes throughout this book to denote the contentious terrain on which it treads. I broadly ascribe to Eric Rofes' argument made in *Dry Bones Breathe* (1998), a book which argues that the mid-to-late 1990s marks a shift in the politics of HIV/AIDS due to the introduction of effective life-extending drugs. I concur with Rofes' argument that while the ongoing nature of the pandemic, especially in the Global South, continues to represent a crisis of significant proportions, the experiences and treatment regimens associated with HIV/AIDS for many in the Global North undoubtedly changed. Indeed, this shift is reflected in my selection of plays and performance works, making Rofes' designation a productive one for my purposes.

of smaller stages in the US and the UK, including London's Trafalgar Studios in 2015. Finally, it would be remiss not to mention Tony Kushner's *Angels in America* (1991), a two-part play whose innumerable revivals and adaptations include an HBO miniseries released in 2003 and sold-out runs at London's National Theatre and Broadway's Neil Simon Theatre between 2017 and 2018.

This chapter argues that such revivals (bar, as we will see, *Angels*) frequently serve conservative hegemonic ends in today's auditoria. While it might be tempting to understand these productions as straightforwardly bestowing historical knowledge upon modern audiences, the decision to continually fund and stage revivals of plays like *The Normal Heart* cannot be isolated from wider ideological forces. As material support for new playwrights grows increasingly threadbare, the channeling of resources into plays that tell thematically analogous stories about the experiences of white, moneyed New Yorkers and their quasi-nuptial relationships during the early AIDS crisis is nothing if not political. The return to decades-old plays is redolent of so-called 'AIDS nostalgia', a cultural fiction that conceptualizes the HIV/AIDS crisis as largely 'over' (at least in the Global North), in large part due to the work of small activist groups in New York and San Francisco. While this highly selective and localized account of history is germane to the creation of digestible cultural commodities for modern audiences, its propagation helps to efface the histories and ongoing realities of constituencies absent from canonized HIV/AIDS plays. Although such work might have served a politically galvanizing purpose when premiered, its continued revival risks producing the opposite effect, cordoning AIDS off as a historical aberration and obscuring how neoliberal governance continues to deny racialized and classed groups of people access to adequate HIV/AIDS healthcare.

Fortunately, awareness of this phenomenon is growing sharply thanks to recent work by a host of scholars, artists, and activists. The recently published edited collection *AIDS and the Distribution of Crises* (2020), for example, asserts the need to understand HIV/AIDS as a cluster of culturally contingent and overlapping crises 'bound up with histories of race, racialization, globalized yet uneven development, and widespread economic inequity' (Cheng et al. 2020, 3). Its chapters cover everything from crises of knowledge production about HIV/AIDS in queer communities of color to the emergence of online AIDS activism. Beyond the realms of academe, visual artists Ian Bradley-Perrin and Vincent Chevalier have critiqued the commodification of HIV/AIDS histories in a poster piece entitled *Your Nostalgia is Killing Me* (2014). The piece portrays what appears to be a teenager's bedroom adorned with Keith Haring wallpaper and posters featuring Gran Fury's iconic "SILENCE=DEATH" slogan, popstar Justin Bieber wearing an ACT UP T-shirt, and an infamous United Colors of Benetton advert featuring a dying AIDS patient. The jarring positioning of commodity culture beside once-dissident protest art highlights how the cooption of AIDS histories by dominant cultural forces has effectively neutralized the politics surrounding the pandemic. Take the "SILENCE=DEATH" iconography as an example. The focal point of the poster is a pink triangle resembling the symbol supposed sexual dissidents were forced to wear in Nazi concentration camps, thus drawing clear comparisons between the genocidal actions of the Nazi regime and the willful inaction of the US government to address AIDS. Since the creation of the image in 1987, however, as Bradley-Perrin explains, its original meaning has been diluted:

> Memories of the significance of this image are not just informed by this moment but are also informed by the years of use and reuse and overuse of this image and are digested not only as memories of the moment but memories of the canonization of the image. When this is told in stories, shared between generations [...] we don't remember its specific claims to genocide [...] It becomes an image of AIDS point finale. (Visual AIDS 2013)

The scores of consumer products emblazoned with Gran Fury's original iconography now sold by corporate giants such as Amazon exemplify how this semiotic shift has occurred. As one Amazon retailer notes in the description of a T-shirt emblazoned with "SILENCE=DEATH," the garment is 'designed for peaceful protest, marches and campaigning against keeping quiet' as well as to 'show your respect and pride for each other', vague and sentimentalized messaging that represents a far cry from the anti-genocidal rhetoric of ACT UP's protests. In purchasing such a T-shirt, then, neoliberal subjects are exhorted to promote themselves as caring and moral individuals through the affective appreciation of a bowdlerized account of history.

Scholars of HIV/AIDS theater are also paying greater attention to the pitfalls of AIDS nostalgia as its depoliticizing effects grow increasingly obvious. Marc Arthur, for example, conceptualizes nostalgic revivals as symptomatic of a heteronormative temporal logic that ignores how the initial 'wounds' of the crisis continue to affect how queer communities live and negotiate intimate relationships, while erroneously creating 'a theatricalized safe distance in which the pain of that period is imbued with desirability' (Arthur 2021, 22). Dirk

Visser, meanwhile, has argued that the hagiographical treatment of Kramer and the continued staging of his work serves to propagate a kind of 'plague rhetoric' that conceptualizes HIV/AIDS as a punishment for promiscuity within gay communities (Visser 2020, 17). In other words, continuing to grant credence to Kramer's puritanical approach to reducing HIV transmission licenses powerful people and institutions to wield stigma as a tool with which to oppress the queer-identified.

While I am sympathetic to these scholarly diagnoses, we cannot avoid the role first-hand loss and grief play in upholding or corroborating certain elements of AIDS nostalgia. As Marika Cifor notes, ACT UP's mobilization of queer community – characterized by consummate examples of care, activism, and cultural production – have shaped contemporary queer identity and politics. Those who dedicated their lives to fighting state neglect

> have a meaningfully distinct longing for ACT UP marked alternately by yearning, grief, anger, and affection. It is in significant part the affective resonances of ACT UP, namely the feeling of queer community and artistically engaged political action across difference, that make it subject and site for nostalgic feelings and memory. (Cifor 2022, 38)

Our task, then, is to disentangle the emotionally fraught and righteous recognition of ACT UP's achievements from AIDS nostalgia's impetus to consign HIV/AIDS to history or redact some of the movement's less auspicious political valences. To achieve this, I tie the normative aspects of AIDS nostalgia to an explicatory framework that takes neoliberal political economy as a prime structuring force motivating the theatrical revivals that resist the potential for self-examination or political reflexivity.

Reviving *The Normal Heart*

Given the relatively substantial number of times Larry Kramer's play has been revived, it represents an apt starting point for untangling how AIDS nostalgia operates as a hegemonic tool of neoliberalism and curtails what we might think of as queer liberationism in a twenty-first-century context. The first production of *The Normal Heart* took place on April 21, 1985 at the Public Theater in New York City. AIDS was sweeping the city's queer communities at the time, and protest movements were still in their relatively nascent stages. Kramer's semi-autobiographical play represented an attempt to raise local consciousness about the scale of the crisis, recounting the early years of the pandemic between 1981 and 1984.

Even before this period, Kramer had made a name for himself as a polemicist opposed to what he saw as gay men's promiscuity and rejection of loving romantic connection. Following a modest career writing plays for stage and screen, he published *Faggots* in 1978 – a novel whose portrayal of gay men's lives in Manhattan was broadly rejected by queer readers as moralistic and aligned with heteronormative politics. In 1981, Kramer got involved in AIDS activism when several friends fell ill, raising funds and providing support services as part of an advocacy group that became known as Gay Men's Health Crisis (GMHC). During this time, he started publishing searing anti-sex essays in popular news outlets and using the stage as a platform from which to proffer didactic messages against promiscuity among gay men. As well as highlighting the inadequacy of AIDS research funding, these activities established Kramer as a divisive and potentially harmful figure in the fight against AIDS, with GMHC ousting him in 1983.[2]

Consistent with his puritanical politics, Kramer crafted *The Normal Heart* as a tragic love story that sees activist Ned (a thinly veiled representation of Kramer himself) forced to witness the death of his closeted lover, Felix. During its first run, this blend of sentimentality and didacticism was used to appeal to both the audience members' political consciences and their empathic capacities. As activist and musician Kevin Robert Frost once recalled in an interview about ACT UP and its legacy, Kramer made clear his motivations for penning the play after meeting Frost in the record shop where the latter worked:

> He was looking for an opera, some obscure opera recording, and I told him I'd help him if we had it. After a few minutes, I finally said to him, *Listen, I just want to tell you that I saw your play,* The Normal Heart, *and it really, really moved me.* And Larry being Larry, looked at me and said, *Oh, that's great. So what the fuck you doin' about it?* (qtd. in Schulman 2021a, 596)

As famously strident in his activism as in his semi-autobiographical playwriting, Kramer's public messaging in all its forms was focused on pushing HIV/AIDS up politicians' agendas, while encouraging regular

2 For a taste of Kramer's polemical style, see "1,112 and Counting," originally published in 1982 (Kramer 2020)

New Yorkers to join the burgeoning ranks of AIDS activists engaging in direct action. Telling real stories about the heroic efforts of activists fighting injustice helped to humanize HIV-positive people at a time when stigma incessantly crushed governmental and societal responses to the crisis. Thanks to images of ACT UP on the news and the creation of cultural products documenting the plight of the infected, the 'new queer/PWA [person with AIDS] stood publicly with power and grace, and the defiant determination had long-range influence on how people with HIV and queer people saw themselves and were in turn understood by others' (Schulman 2021a, 9). Kramer's play contributed to this shift in cultural common sense, even garnering sympathetic responses from the *New York Times,* whose coverage of the early years of the AIDS crisis has been heavily critiqued as stigmatizing by activists and scholars alike. As one critic noted of the initial production, while 'Mr. Kramer's theatrical talents are not always as highly developed as his conscience, there can be little doubt that *The Normal Heart* is the most outspoken play around – or that it speaks up about a subject that justifies its author's unflagging, at times even hysterical, sense of urgency' (Rich 1985).

As well as directly targeting the pharmaceutical and governmental powers that held HIV-positive people hostage through flagrant denial of material support, activists operating in the era before protease inhibitors intuited the importance of cultural engagement in achieving their goals.[3] Figures such as Kramer might be conceptualized – in Gramscian military parlance – as 'the leading personnel, and of what may be called the "front-line" (and assault) forces' in 'the strategic preparation of the theatre of struggle' (Gramsci 2003, 217). In exploiting the affective capacities of those otherwise alienated from struggle on the ground, the work of artists and activists weakened phobic attitudes toward non-normative sexualities and passive consent for the mistreatment of people with HIV, helping to put into motion political decisions that eventually facilitated the production of life-saving treatments. While Kramer's anti-sex messaging was problematic in various ways, his brash and unrelenting approach to both his activism and artistic work reflect an assiduous commitment to preventing further loss of life – even if it meant putting his reputation

3 Protease inhibitors are medications that prevent HIV from replicating and are often used in combination with other drugs to manage HIV. They were approved for use in 1995 and continue to comprise treatment regimens for people living with HIV today. Some protease inhibitors are also used to treat other viral infections, including hepatitis C and COVID-19.

and personal relationships on the line. Given the cultural purchase enjoyed at the time by homophobic political constituencies, Kramer's interventions represented vital weapons with which to wrest back control of cultural narratives.

For all the good that can be attributed to *The Normal Heart*, however, the function of its sentimentalized and didactic anti-sex messaging has inevitably grown more vulnerable to critique in line with conjunctural shifts. Take, by way of example, a rather lengthy speech made by protagonist Ned following his expulsion from the activist organization he helped to create. He asserts his belonging to a culture that includes (among many others listed) Proust, Socrates, Christopher Marlowe, Lorca, E.M. Forster, and Alan Turing. Lauding these men as exemplars of the strength of gay men, he goes on:

> The only way we'll have real pride is when we demand recognition of a culture that isn't just sexual. It's all there – all through history we've been there; but we have to claim it, and identify who was in it, and articulate what's in our minds and hearts and all our creative contributions to this earth. And until we do that, and until we organize ourselves block by neighborhood by city by state into a united visible community that fights back, we're doomed. That's how I want to be defined: as one of the men who fought the war. Being defined by our cocks is literally killing us. (Kramer 2011, 70–1)

Such rhetoric might have served a practical purpose at the time, given the life-or-death exigencies of New York's 'crisis years'. While Kramer's anti-sex message was no doubt controversial in activist circles, particularly given the incremental gains gay liberation movements had only recently won, there's no denying that reducing sexual contact represents a practical approach to lowering viral transmission rates. However, its teleological appeal to a kind of bounded community with a noble history driven by 'elders' represents an essentialist approach to sexual politics that figures his gayness as fixed, rather than a category shaped by (and actively involved in the renegotiation of) hegemonic standards.

As we will explore in greater depth in later chapters, such a view has been repeatedly undermined as politically limited and historically illiterate thanks to the work of queer theorists influenced by variously materialist and Foucauldian understandings of power, domination, and the development of social norms. At the most basic level, to label Socrates or Christopher Marlowe as 'gay' is to erroneously project contemporary understandings of sexual identity onto historical moments in which notions such as heterosexuality or homosexuality were yet to take shape. In fudging the complex, contingent, and contested histories of sexuality in this way, Kramer naturalizes a hetero–homo binary that views an oppressed 'gay community' as at 'war' with power-wielding straights. As clarified by Ned's speeches surrounding the powers of love and monogamy, his perceived logical way to overcome such inequity is to fight for subsumption into already existing socio-economic structures and institutions (such as marriage).

What this view overlooks, of course, are the ways in which this subsumption gives tacit consent to oppressive structures. The subject of gay marriage, while often cited as the lynchpin of gay liberation in mainstream left-liberal and centrist political discourse, has long been cited by queer and feminist academics as a paragon of *homonormativity*. Coined by Lisa Duggan in her turn-of-the-millennium study of neoliberalism, *The Twilight of Equality?* (2003), homonormativity betrays 'a politics that does not contest dominant heteronormative assumptions and institutions, but upholds and sustains them, while promising the possibility of a demobilized gay constituency and a privatized, depoliticized gay culture anchored in domesticity and consumption' (Duggan 2003, 50). Gay proponents of homonormativity thus express a desire for subjection to neoliberal governance and for acceptance by a 'national mainstream', serving to drive 'a rhetorical remapping of public/private boundaries designed to shrink gay public spheres, and redefine gay equality against the "civil rights agenda" and "liberationism," as access to the institutions of domestic privacy, the "free" market, and patriotism' (Duggan 2003, 50–1). More recently, Stephen Valocchi has observed that neoliberalism's continued decimation of state assistance for the poor has revealed marriage to be a form of coercive 'risk management' for couples of all orientations due to the social and financial benefits tied to legally recognized matrimony (Valocchi 2020, 151–2). As such, materially disadvantaged queers are incentivized to adopt homonormative structures as a means to mitigate the risk of future destitution. By devoting themselves entirely to each other and adopting homo/heteronormative traditions, Ned and Felix tacitly (perhaps unknowingly) enter into a contract with the neoliberal state. While the protagonists' incursion into heterosexual legal structures might have seemed radical and bellicose on the first showing of *The Normal Heart*, the couple's domestication ultimately takes on different connotations in contemporary contexts.

So, how do theaters and those involved in productions of the play navigate this tension? And why do some of the world's most influential theaters tend to prioritize the staging of early HIV/AIDS plays to the exclusion of more recent works (such as those explored in the later chapters of this book)? I am wary of painting the revival of older plays as inevitably nostalgic, regressive, or reactionary here – there may be, after all, value in examining Kramer's text as illustrative of a particular moment in the history of HIV/AIDS activism. In portraying the harsh realities experienced by HIV-positive people of earlier generations, the play has the potential to deepen the empathetic capacities of younger toward older queer people (and indeed between otherwise marginalized constituencies), building critical camaraderie at a time when threats to queer communities and lifeways are far from over. We might continue to learn from previous political movements, applying their practical and tactical lessons to an updated social and political context. At the same time, the potential for plays like *The Normal Heart* to deliver a sense of affirmation for people with HIV should not be underestimated, providing recognition and solidarity in sincere and discerning forms.

At a broader level, however, the continued appraisal of *The Normal Heart* as 'timely and essential' (Curtis 2021), combined with the inadequately critical historicization of the play by those involved in its revival, mean AIDS nostalgia lives on. In a promotional video for the 2021 production at London's National Theatre, for example, Elander Moore (a young actor who played Craig Donner) describes his appreciation of the play as an elucidatory polemic that teaches young people about queer history and the groups of activists to whom they can attribute their relative sexual freedom, thus reinscribing Kramer's politically limited teleology (National Theatre 2021). Having not been taught queer history in school, he suggests, productions of plays such as *The Normal Heart* play an important role in helping queer youth understand their heritage and, indeed, themselves. While there is certainly a kernel of truth in Moore's words regarding the dearth of queer history on school syllabi, we have already seen that the unquestioning acceptance of gayness as grounded in kinship has political limitations. What's more, the play's exaltation of affective display as a galvanizing tool in and of itself has perversely depoliticizing effects in a culture where the neoliberalization of the self permeates both ends of the political spectrum.

To clarify what I mean by this, I turn briefly to Dirk Gindt's essay 'National Performances of Crying: Neoliberal Sentimentality and the Cultural Commodification of HIV and AIDS in Sweden' (2018), which casts a critical eye over the interaction between social media and marketable cultural products, while using such participatory platforms to gauge how audiences receive HIV/AIDS theater in the twenty-first century. Gindt provides an analysis of how digital culture influences the ways in which early HIV/AIDS plays are adapted for a contemporary audience, homing in on how Swedish playwright Jonas Gardell reshaped his 1989 play *Ömheten* [*Tenderness*] for a 2012 television series entitled *Torka aldrig tårar utan handskar* [*Don't Ever Wipe Tears Without Gloves*], as well as an onstage revival by Stockholm City Theatre in the same year. These newer versions depart from the original play in ways that adhere to nostalgic imperatives. For example, Rasmus and Benjamin (the story's coupled-up protagonists) have an open relationship in *Ömheten*, and Rasmus is exposed to HIV during a casual hookup. In the 2012 version, however, Rasmus is seropositive when he meets Benjamin, having been exposed to HIV during his very first sexual encounter. It also contains a deathbed scene complete with AIDS nostalgia's tell-tale quasi-nuptial tropes, signaling that the couple have 'overcome' what Kramer so often pathologized as the sex-obsessed impulsiveness of gay hookup culture.

The decision to imbue Gardell's newer plays with more nostalgic tropes might be understood as exemplary of what Akane Kanai and Rosalind Gill conceptualize as 'woke capitalism'. Although I am wary of deploying the term 'woke' in this context, particularly given its weaponization by rightward forces to attack even moderate moves toward social justice reform, Kanai and Gill's formulation helps elucidate how financial interests support the production of *seemingly* counterhegemonic or liberationist cultural products that actually rigidify exploitative ideologies. Asserting that affect's hegemonic role has been left undertheorized in Gramscian conjunctural analysis, the pair theorize woke capitalism as a structuring force that not only *reflects* dominant values, but 'produces a particular imaginary through the *disarticulation and rearticulation* of social struggle and emancipatory utopias' (Kanai and Gill 2020, 21, emphasis in original). In line with neoliberalism's atomizing imperatives, woke capitalist cultural products and organizations are invested in neat narratives of 'overcoming', whereby embodying a position as a 'marginalised, excluded and highly surveilled subject is translated as a *personal* injury, thus making racial, gendered, and sexualised oppression a matter of individual responsibility and attitudinal orientation' (Kanai and Gill 2020, 23, emphasis in original). Examples provided include Beyonce's visual album *Black is King* (2020), conceptualized as a 'love letter' to the African diaspora and a personal narrative of inspirational overcoming on the popstar's journey to international fame. As Kanai and Gill point out, this individualist approach to addressing inequity casts non-dominant people as 'visible, neoliberal subjects of potential value, their historical experiences of oppression intertwined with an associated generalised sense of positivity, possibility, belief in capitalist futurity, and commitment to self-work' (Kanai and Gill 2020, 24). Similarly, the promotion of Gardell's play as 'the all-inclusive and definitive history of AIDS in Sweden' (Gindt 2018, 248) and a nostalgic story in which minoritarian subjects 'explode expectations' in the face of hardship places it comfortably within the category of woke capitalism.

In characterizing the couple as monogamous and Rasmus's exposure as the product of (later conquered) youthful folly, the 2012 play and TV series thus hail the normative sensibilities of the neoliberal subject while encouraging viewers to identify themselves with the play's central protagonists. As Gindt explains, the commercial brains behind these cultural products encouraged very public outpourings of emotion via online forums, appealing to the individualistic impulse that undergirds woke capitalism. To back up this claim, he conducted an extensive Twitter search using the hashtag #torkaaldrigtårar, observing that social media became a ground for competitive testimonies of weeping, sparking 'a competition of who would cry more, faster and better' (Gindt 2018, 247). He also notes that

> The twenty-first century neoliberal subjects tweeting or posting their affective responses were grounding their emotional self-identification in vague notions of 'tolerance' and 'diversity' and a combination of sentimentality and nostalgia rather than a critical investigation of how the AIDS epidemic of the past continues to influence contemporary mechanisms of sexual regulation, HIV policy and stigmatisation. (Gindt 2018, 248)

The television production and revival of the play, then, encouraged viewers to ignore the ways in which HIV/AIDS remains a political issue by exploiting a desire for sentimentalized narratives uncomplicated by the serpentine political terrain people with HIV are forced to navigate in the present. Rather than increasing awareness of issues surrounding, say, legislation and stigma, the process of revival offers ample opportunity for neoliberal subjects to lament the political missteps of the past through affective posturing that functions as a kind of productive work designed to boost likes, shares, and a personal 'brand'.

While it is easy to dismiss social platforms as innocuous forums through which theatergoers can share their opinions, such platforms play an increasingly important role in the promotion of cultural products. Displays of online affect that attest to a play's emotional power and impressive stylistics might encourage the original poster's friends or acquaintances to purchase tickets, thereby generating revenue for the theater venue and bolstering the reputations of those involved with the creation of the work. The posters themselves might also personally benefit from their Tweets or messages (however mawkish), as they serve to cultivate the personal 'brand' demanded by the tacit mechanisms of neoliberal hegemony. As Richard Seymour notes in his cautionary polemic, *The Twittering Machine* (2019), the digital revolution has intensified some of neoliberalism's most anti-communitarian psychosocial pathologies. Enmeshed in a culture where the 'online self' has become a necessary appendage for developing social and financial capital, the social network 'compels us to dedicate more and more of our time to performing an identity [...] We can carefully brand ourselves, producing an identity as a consumable good, an attention magnet' (Seymour 2019, 100). In this way, websites such as Twitter and Facebook provide convenient forums for cultural consumers to comment on plays, artworks, or films by allowing users to conduct affective displays as vehicles for self-promotion.

Despite the obviously shaky ethical terrain on which HIV/AIDS theater revivals stand, I approach Gindt's analysis with a degree of caution. The producers of Broadway's 2011 production of *The Normal Heart*, for example, made sure to gesture toward the continued urgency of the pandemic. In fact, Isaac West has argued that – contrary to the conceptualization of *The Normal Heart* as a relic of its time and a document of the crisis years – its 2011 revival constituted an effective piece of educational and activist theater. By 'emphasizing the play's non-fictional nature and evoking compassion and sympathy, it reinforced the gravity of the subject matter by reminding the audience that HIV/AIDS impacts real people, now as it did then' (West 2012, 100). One of the main ways in which this was achieved, West posits, was through the distribution of a letter to audience members penned by Kramer himself, headed 'PLEASE KNOW'. In it, Kramer makes the following entreaty to the audience:

> Please know that there is no one in charge of this plague. This is a war for which there is no general and for which there has never been a general. How can you win a war with no one in charge?
>
> Please know that beginning with Ronald Reagan (who would not say the word 'AIDS' publicly for seven years), every single president has said nothing and done nothing, or in the case of the current president [Obama], says the right things and then doesn't do them.
>
> Please know that most medications for HIV/AIDS are inhumanly

> expensive and that government funding for the poor to obtain them is dwindling and often unavailable. (Kramer 2011, 79)

In acknowledging HIV/AIDS as an ongoing crisis in the US and setting out a genealogy of presidential apathy in relation to the disease, Kramer attempts to offset tendencies toward nostalgia and emphasize the importance of productive public conversation surrounding the virus. However, as West concedes, 'Kramer does not direct the audience to take any particular action and leaves it up to them how best to direct their emotional energy' (West 2012, 101).

A quick Twitter search, following Gindt's methodology, gives us some idea of the way in which such emotional energy is spent. US news anchor Don Lemon, for example, watched the show and tweeted, in a similar tone to that employed by Gindt's Swedish Twitter subjects, 'What an incredible show & cast. so emotional. i'm dehydrated from crying so much. wow. larry was there too' (@donlemon), while another audience member explained how '@thenormalheart hit my conscious with a sledgehammer and demolished me into a sobbing mess. Pls learn more about HIV/AIDS: www.aids.gov' (@DeanneChen). By suggesting that he experienced a painful somatic reaction – dehydration – to Kramer's play, Lemon attempts to sell himself as a model empathic agent: someone so affected by the plight of the AIDS-afflicted that he feels physical pain. While he might indeed have experienced a feeling of genuine empathy, the possibility that this feeling was interpenetrated by self-promotional desires is only made more plausible by the jarring statement 'larry was there too'. This phrase betrays a valorization of celebrity consistent with hierarchical neoliberal logic, as well as the fact that as a well-known public figure himself, Lemon has a strong imperative to sell himself to an audience base. The author of the latter tweet, meanwhile, turns attention toward their own capacity for self-betterment with a comically hyperbolic sledgehammer metaphor. The shattering of the misapplied term 'conscious' implies the total destruction of an aspect of their worldview that we can assume is undesirable or unenlightened, making way for cognitive reparations to make them a better person. Consistent with woke capitalism's narrative of 'overcoming', their entreaty to followers to learn more about HIV/AIDS via an official US government website conceptualizes the ongoing pandemic as the product of a citizenry's psychic deficits, rather than the failings of the dominant powers that Kramer's play excoriates.

Such hyperbolic testimonies, then, in their sheer ferocity and inward-looking focus on their authors' emotional responses, support

Gindt's thesis that the revival of HIV/AIDS plays can instigate competitive displays of affect that contain little to no counterhegemonic substance. In a conjuncture characterized by social atomism and the incursion of individualist logic into the very fabric of contemporary lived experience, restaging decades-old plays inevitably generates very different cultural interventions compared to their original productions. In laying historicist claim to an 'official' narrative of HIV/AIDS in the Global North surrounding grassroots 'overcoming', nostalgic plays overlook the experiences of people marginalized on several counts (their gender, race, class etc.), while (however inadvertently) satisfying the woke capitalist imperatives of a liberal milieu affectively attached to individualistic diversity rhetoric. What this calls for, I argue, is a greater appreciation for capitalism's historical role in perpetuating the stigmatization and malignant neglect of people living with HIV. While many of the more popular older HIV/AIDS plays categorically fail in this regard, others continue to present potentially valuable materialist interventions. Next, then, I will explore one of the genre's more forthrightly socialistic early works.

Angels in America: a critical reappraisal

Tony Kushner's *Angels in America* presents a few challenges to the picture I have painted of HIV/AIDS play revivals and their often-contradictory politics. Unlike other early plays that focused primarily on the lives of gay couples affected by the virus, Kushner painted a picture of the epidemic that transcended the experiences of its central protagonists, HIV-positive Prior and his partner Louis, who leaves Prior following his AIDS diagnosis. With a combined run-time approaching eight hours, both parts of *Angels* use the central theme of disease to explore not only the impact of HIV/AIDS on people's lives, but themes reflecting the wider US political arena of the time – the cruelties of Reaganomics, global warming, culture wars, America's religious landscape, and the enduring legacy of McCarthyism, to name but a few. On the one hand, reactions to the play's recent revivals in London and New York demonstrate its nostalgic potential, generating affective outpourings about Prior and Louis's relationship being 'fundamentally about forgiveness and human connections [...] quiet heroism and healing' (Rooney 2018), echoing reactions to *The Normal Heart* and *Torka aldrig tårar utan handskar*.

Such sentimental responses should come as no surprise given the playtext's more platitudinous lines, many of which gesture toward teleological rationalisms that align with the neat triumphalism of AIDS nostalgia. The epilogue, for example – in which protagonists Prior, Louis, Belize, and Hannah directly address the audience several years after the pandemic has touched their lives – contains ostensibly quixotic or millenarian accounts of the future, such as Louis's 'That's what politics is. The world moving ahead. And only in politics does the miraculous occur'; Hannah's 'The fountain of Bethesda will flow again [...] We will all bathe ourselves clean'; and, most famously, Prior's 'The world only spins forward. We will be citizens. The time has come' (Kushner [1993] 2017, 288–90). It cannot be denied, furthermore, that the play centers on the interests of moneyed white men orbited by a cast of women and people of color, each of whom spends at least some of their time attending to the men's emotional and physical needs. In so doing, it might be read as playing into hegemonic stereotypes counterintuitive to a liberatory politics capable of critiquing oppression across difference.

However, Kushner's play consistently presents counterarguments to undermine the nostalgic impulses of its characters, demonstrating its alignment with an anti-capitalist, socialistic politics that does not *necessarily* propagate an assimilative view of gay kinship. Shot through with references to Walter Benjamin's revolutionary treatise, 'Theses on the Philosophy of History' (1942), *Angels* looks beyond its protagonists' personal concerns to present a long rumination about political organization on the left, invoking historical materialist theories to consider how life could be improved for queer, HIV-positive, and other marginalized people in ways glaringly absent from other plays of its stature. Despite its dated setting, *Angels* continues to raise questions about the continued failings of liberal democracy – seen, for example, in the parallels between Roy Cohn and contemporary right-wing Americans such as Trump, as well as the current deepening of the ecological crisis upon which Harper fixates. In so doing, it reveals a structure of feeling more closely aligned to a universalist politics of HIV/AIDS than might first appear. Using *Angels* and its legacy as an example, I will show how AIDS nostalgia is potentially avoidable on the neoliberal stage under the right conditions and directorship. While Kushner's play is by no means straightforwardly counterhegemonic, its contradictions, ambiguities, and revolutionary spirit lay the introductory groundwork for a Gramscian critique of contemporary HIV/AIDS theater, which will aid discussion of lesser-known plays and performances in the later chapters of this book.

When unearthing the counterhegemonic potentialities of *Angels*, it is worth paying heed to critiques of the more nostalgic (or arguably anti-liberatory) elements of the play's politics. By countering critical analyses that overlook what I consider the play's epistemic humility in this way, one can begin to unveil how *Angels* doubles up as a theoretical text interested in the role of the dialectic for understanding histories of oppression – and a warning against the dangers of teleological historicist approaches (to which AIDS nostalgia so clearly falls victim). For some scholars, the dualities and ambiguities threaded throughout *Angels* represent both a source of frustration and evidence of a hidden conservativism. David Savran, for example, offered one of the earliest theoretical critiques of the play's anti-capitalist credentials in the mid-1990s, arguing that its counterhegemonic dramaturgies are compromised by an attachment to a kind of American liberal pluralism that valorizes identitarian forms of politics at the expense of the play's materialist imperatives. Analyzing the character of Louis (who, he argues, is the 'most empathic character in the play', despite abandoning his dying lover), Savran notes that his outspoken faith in some kind of radical liberal democracy assures the theatergoing public that gradualist reform remains the best organizing force for change. Many of Louis's arguments with sparring partner Belize revolve around the role of race and gender in America, with the former arguing that increasingly liberal social attitudes are improving the lives of all. Thus, 'revolution, in the Marxist sense, is rendered virtually unthinkable, oxymoronic. Amidst all the political disputation, there is no talk of social class. Oppression is understood not in relation to economics but to differences of race, gender and sexual orientation' (Savran 1995, 214). Here, Savran appears dissatisfied with the play's infidelities to a (now largely discredited) strand of orthodox Marxism, the rigid economism of which leaves little room to theorize how categories like race and class might interact. In so doing, he ignores or works against swathes of what might variously be termed post-Marxist, New Left, or Black Marxist scholarship by the likes of, say, C.L.R. James, Cedric Robinson, or indeed Antonio Gramsci, each of whom wrote about how categories such as race were deployed and naturalized to shore up capitalism's position as the dominant economic order.

While Savran characterizes Louis's interactions with Belize as indicative of the play's lack of anti-capitalist consciousness, I view them as a lens through which to understand how oppression is meted out under a sociopolitical order built on a fiction of equal opportunities and meritocracy. Although I sympathize with the impulse to critique Kushner for his unwillingness to commit to an ideological schema grounded in socialistic justice, the play's sprawling text and the characters who inhabit its diegesis appear clearly, at times self-reflexively, flawed and politically illiterate by design. Contradicting Savran's characterization as the play's most 'empathic' character, for example, Louis rambles in a confused fashion about race and identity, exclaiming,

> Racists just try to use race here as a tool in political struggle. It's not really about race. Like the spiritualists try to use that stuff, are you enlightened, are you centered, channeled, whatever, this reaching out for a spiritual past in a country where no indigenous spirits exist – only the Indians, I mean Native American spirits and we killed them off so now, there are no gods here, no ghosts and spirits in America, there are no angels in America, no spiritual past, no racial past, there's only the political, and the decoys and the ploys to maneuver around the inescapable battle of politics, the shifting downwards and outwards of political power to the people—. (Kushner [1993] 2017, 104)

Such an argument represents the antithesis of a historical materialist reading of America's political landscape, revealing an utter disregard for the material bases on which the oppression of marginalized groups (including, of course, HIV-positive people) have been built over decades and centuries. Interpenetrating this sprawling rant is a parallel scene (typically staged side-by-side), in which Prior strips naked to unveil a host of new lesions to his nurse. This image provides a visceral and visual counterpoint to the idealist notions of political progress put forward by Louis, who has not borne the brunt of the horrors inflicted by Reaganite governance in the US and, perhaps tellingly, confesses to possessing a 'neo-Hegelian positivist sense of constant progress towards happiness or perfection or something' early on in the play (Kushner [1993] 2017, 25). His statement that there are no 'ghosts' haunting America elides the ways in which centuries of expropriative colonialism and neocolonialism undermine this claim to 'progress', as the unbridled accumulation of wealth that blooms from such plunder continues to deepen inequalities that negatively affect the already racialized and stigmatized. The experiential gap between those Americans suffering (i.e., Prior) and those around them (i.e., Louis), who are free to simply intellectualize the nature of such misery, as Stephanie Byttebier has observed, foregrounds 'the enormous difficulty of solidarity in a world replete with suffering' (Byttebier 2011, 289), pushing audience members to think beyond vacuous axioms of solidarity and progress to consider more difficult questions about how the suffering with which they are confronted can be addressed or even palliated in tangible ways.

For Savran, Kushner's drift away from neat economic analyses of class domination betrays an outlook that 'unabashedly champions rationalism and progress' and remains the product of an idealist, gradualist politics lacking the counterhegemonic power to realize a world beyond neoliberal America (Savran 1995, 214). However, as Roger Bechtel explains in an essay rebutting Savran's claims, it is important to understand *Angels* in its late twentieth-century context before condemning its lack of classical Marxist analysis or failure to offer hope of seismic political revolution. Such expectations betray a kind of nostalgia for theories no longer applicable to a contemporary political landscape that Kushner quite rightly views as lacking a cohesive politics of the left, so eroded has it been by the common sense of neoliberal hegemony. Indeed, 'what Kushner grapples with in his play is the very problem of effecting political praxis in the absence of theory; in a world where Marxism is struggling against its widely-perceived death-blow, realpolitik requires rethinking traditional approaches to "revolution"' (Bechtel 2001, 102). Of course, revolutionary strategy is a notoriously fraught point of contention within wider Marxist and socialist traditions, with Western Marxist thinkers more than willing to break from the formulaic orthodoxies of classical Marxism. *Angels*, in some ways, can be seen to represent a reflection on revolutionary heterodoxies in an increasingly capitalistic twentieth century, with its vigorous yet ambivalent revolutionary spirit containing something of a Gramscian consciousness – committed as Gramsci was to formulating a coherent theory of revolution against a historical backdrop marred by factional crises within the Western European left and the encroaching threat of fascism.

To clarify, Gramsci's discussion of revolution in *The Prison Notebooks* was interested in the temporal relation between theory and struggle on the ground. As Fabio Frosini notes, Gramsci viewed historiography as playing a vital role in the grammar of political movements, allowing counterhegemonic forces to critically interpret and reinterpret the present as determined by past events. Indeed, 'the victories (or defeats) of the past reaffirm themselves in the present thanks to historical accounts, while the conflicting critical and strategic elaborations realized by the forces in struggle help these to "resolve" the conflict in one or another direction' (Frosini 2019, 125). If such a relationship is mediated dialectically, a so-called 'permanent revolution' might result (i.e., a productive break toward a socialistic organization of society). If, on the other hand, one carries out a simple 'deduction' from the conflict between past and present, that is, 'when a class of intellectuals succeeds in "absorbing" within its own discourse the political dimension of the class struggle', an anti-liberationist 'passive revolution' might result – which, as Frosini notes, represents a type of hegemony (Frosini 2019, 138–9). Indeed, the aforementioned problematic of 'woke capitalism' might be seen as exemplary of such passive revolution, whereby institutions and political structures incrementally mutate to quash growing discontentment toward overtly discriminatory practices of the ruling classes, without their having to relinquish significant power or capital.

Angels is similarly interested in the incursion of the past on contemporaneous political struggle and how historical knowledge might be deployed in dialectical conflict. Take the representation of Roy Cohn, a character who (while partly fictionalized) is largely based on the real-life history of his infamous namesake. Outside the world of the play, Cohn is best known for his role in the Army–McCarthy hearings, during which he successfully prosecuted communists Julius and Ethel Rosenberg for espionage, leading to their executions in 1953. Cohn's death has also courted attention over the years, the liver cancer from which he reportedly suffered clearly a fiction concocted to cover his AIDS diagnosis and sexual past. In *Angels*, Ethel Rosenberg returns as a ghost (or, at least, a kind of vivid illusion) to taunt Roy as he slowly dies of AIDS. While interacting with the play's non-spectral characters, Roy's commitment to a kind of ruthlessly individualistic and Hobbesian conservatism is unwavering:

> My generation, we had *clarity*. Unafraid to look deep into the miasma at the heart of the world, what a pit, what a nightmare is there – *I* have looked, I have searched all my life for absolute bottom, and I found it, *believe* me: *Stygian*. How tragic, how brutal life is. How false people are. The immutable heart of what we are that bleeds through whatever we might become. All else is vanity. (Kushner [1993] 2017, 210)

Such philosophical surety aligns with the kind of Cold War triumphalism that animated dominant discourses surrounding the apparent victory of global capitalism over communist alternatives, best summed up by Francis Fukuyama's (now largely discredited) 'end of history' thesis. Unable to countenance capitalism's failure, Roy believes the essentially exploitative nature of human character might as well realize its intended apotheosis.

With this in mind, a kind of philosophical tussle emerges through Ethel's return. Roy is rattled by her appearance and its implication, to the extent that he deigns to ask Belize, who he spends much of the play taunting and belittling, for his opinions on the existence of heaven and hell. Roy spends the final moments of his life in the company of Ethel, who is exposed to the pain and degradation AIDS inflicts on the bodies of the infected. At first, she feels nothing but a vengeful pleasure in Roy's pain, stating:

> I came to forgive but all I can do is take pleasure in your misery. Hoping I'd get to see you die more terrible than I did. And you are, 'cause you're dying in shit, Roy, defeated. And you could kill me, but you couldn't ever defeat me. You never won. And when you die all anyone will say is: Better he had never lived at all. (Kushner [1993] 2017, 253)

During the McCarthy era, of course, people who engaged in same-sex relations were deemed deviant threats to American domestic security, equal to immigrants and communists in their supposed immorality or perversions. Thanks in part to the ways in which Cold War psychiatrists pathologized non-normative sexual behaviors, many employees of the State Department saw themselves dismissed for 'immoral conduct' (Genter 2017, 1093), illustrating the fragile ground on which Cohn's double life rested. In seeing the shit-soaked consequences of what would have been considered Roy's 'deviancy' during and even beyond the McCarthy era, Ethel gains a kind of moral primacy over her former prosecutor. Having learned that she and Roy would have been classed as similarly threatening and depraved during the hearings, Ethel takes pleasure in their relationship's altered dynamic – Roy's suffering representing a kind of *quid pro quo* for the suffering he inflicted on her.

Here, both characters stand in for something much larger than themselves: Ethel the spirit of a communistic politics increasingly smothered and besmirched under neoliberal orthodoxy; Roy the instantiation of a Hobbesian ruthlessness foundational to late capitalism. Ethel's claim to undefeatability in the face of Roy metaphorizes the ongoing struggle between broadly defined capitalistic and communistic tendencies. However futile or downtrodden anti-capitalist movements might have appeared in the mid-90s, characterized as this era was by the enthusiastic belief in a heuristic 'end of history', Ethel's insight into Roy's vulnerability hints toward the hope that wider hegemonic forces might not be as rock-solid as they first appear. In this instance and throughout *Angels*, capitalism is haunted by the threat of communistic consciousness and the possibility of what Benjamin termed a 'messianic cessation of happening' – a rupture in the existing dominant order that might allow the historical materialist and revolutionary to 'blast a specific era out of the homogenous course of history' and in so doing 'blast open the continuum of history' (Benjamin [1968] 2015, 254).

Later in the scene, however, this revolutionary optimism is tempered by Kushner's characteristic ambivalence. Feigning sudden cognitive incapacitation, Roy pretends to believe that Ethel is his mother and cries about feeling scared. She takes pity on him and gives in to his requests that she sing him a song to relieve the pain. After she sings to him in Yiddish, Roy quickly snaps out of his act and boasts that it is he who can claim victory in their decades-long feud: 'I fooled you, Ethel! I knew who you were all along! I can't believe you fell for that Ma stuff!! I just wanted to see if I could finally, *finally* make Ethel Rosenberg sing! *I WIN!*' (Kushner [1993] 2017, 255). A moment of potential harmony or commonality is immediately quashed, demonstrating again Byttebier's point about solidarity's impossibility in the face of such suffering. Seconds later, Roy is dead, and Ethel is left without having had the final word. After watching Louis struggle to recite the Kaddish next to Roy's body (a favor for Belize), Ethel calls Roy a 'sonofabitch' and vanishes, never to reappear on stage. Assuming again that Ethel and Roy's antagonistic relationship represents larger political struggles, communism's flickering spirit is, for now, extinguished. Failure and ideological impasses, we learn, are an inevitable part of revolutionary struggle. In the wider context of the play, therefore, it falls on other (non-spectral) characters to drive its internal dialectic forward, most notably in the epilogue.

This final scene is set next to the Bethesda Fountain in New York's Central Park, with Belize, Hannah, Louis, and Prior debating world affairs ranging from the fall of the Berlin Wall to the Israeli–Palestinian conflict. Although disagreement reigns, the group experiences revelatory, politically productive moments of realization and solidarity throughout the short scene. When Louis equates politics with a kind of miraculous, idealist progress, for example, Belize challenges the purely theoretical nature of his claim. Hannah then chimes in, resolving this antagonism by explaining that 'You can't live in the world without an idea of the world, but it's the living that makes the ideas. You can't wait for a theory, but you have to have a theory' (Kushner [1993] 2017, 289). As Bechtel explains, rather than resting on the idealist epistemologies Savran detects in *Angels*, such instances of debate and resolution actually reflect Kushner's unwillingness to commit to a grand narrative or bounded, unified theory. Instead, the play puts forward a 'non-theory' of interconnectedness driven by 'a praxis of plurality that will, in dialectical fashion, generate its own theory' (Bechtel 2001, 117–18). By dint of the play's commitment to an ongoing dialectic, then, Louis and Belize soon move on to new heated arguments after Hannah resolves their prior antagonism, something which helps to generate new and productive ways of thinking politically. It is in such moments when the dialectic freezes that Bechtel identifies a 'momentary picture of coalition [in which] we can imagine an articulated counterhegemony of the left' (Bechtel 2001, 118).

Similarly, for David Román, this praxis of plurality is exemplified by the generation of the 'new kinship structure' which Prior, Louis, Belize and Hannah comprise, along with its deviation from 'heteronormative reproductive family structures' (Román 1998, 213). This is because the process of building such bonds of kinship is shown to reflect the enduring dialectic Bechtel theorizes, with each changing their political worldview over time as they are confronted with their complicity in oppressive or dysfunctional social alliances:

> For Prior, this involves an extensive working through and subsequent rejection of the teleology of angelology and a restructuring of his relationship with Louis; for Belize, it involves a confirmation of the powers of love in the midst of racial hatred and oppression; for Hannah Pitt, it involves a deliberate divorce from the orthodoxy of heteronormativity; and for Louis, the journey transforms his positivist concept of history into a more direct responsibility toward the "time of the now." (Román 1998, 213)

In this way, *Angels* laid a kind of blueprint for counterhegemonic political organization for implementation outside the confines of the auditorium. Certainly, Prior's direct address to the audience, in which he pronounces that 'The Great Work Begins', the final line of the play, strongly supports this notion, encouraging the formation of counterhegemonic coalitions across identitarian boundaries to engage in the kinds of dialectical work that Kushner conceives as progress (Kushner [1993] 2017, 290). It also, perhaps, represents a kind of Brechtian dramaturgical blueprint for creators of HIV/AIDS plays hoping to surmount the neoliberal imperatives of the contemporary theatrical institution.

Having gone some way toward addressing Savran's claims surrounding *Angels'* (lack of) theoretical value, then, it would be remiss not to wrap up this chapter without mentioning critiques of the play's more practical political implications. Some take issue with the lessons mainstream contemporary audiences might derive from *Angels*, particularly those who might not be *au fait* with Marxist theory or, indeed, the politics of the AIDS crisis. For example, Schulman's assessment in *Let the Record Show* (2021), one of the most detailed accounts of ACT UP's complex history, is less interested in a philosophy of praxis and more concerned with what the play's individual characters represent, filtered as her view is through her experiences as an activist. The play's storyline, Schulman argues, in which a gay man dying of AIDS is abandoned by his lover and later 'saved' by the straight, homophobic, Mormon mother of his ex-lover's closeted boyfriend misrepresents the realities of the crisis on the ground. Contrary to such a narrative, 'gay men with AIDS were abandoned by most straight people including their families, neighbors, and government. And they were defended by their community, who often shared their lack of rights and representation' (Schulman 2021a, xx).

To make matters worse, Schulman goes on, Kushner's play ends on a note of hope symbolized by the drug azidothymidine (AZT), which was considered lethal by many AIDS activists (who were 'the real hope for the future') by the time of the play's opening (Schulman 2021a, xx). Although *Angels* is set a little earlier in the crisis, when AZT was still considered promising, it is certainly true that representing the drug as potentially curative could offer unhelpful messaging to theatergoers. However, the idea that it is the moral obligation of playwrights to accurately represent the history of a heterogeneous (and often internally conflictual) milieu of AIDS activist groups is both practically unworkable and antithetical to the universalistic politics necessary for addressing the crisis beyond the confines of white, gay America. Strategically, Schulman's approach assumes a non-dialectical, pedagogic relationship between the play and its audience, with the former designed to feed information to the latter. The notion that enlightening viewers in such a way is enough to effect change on the ground promotes idealist modes of thinking over materialist politics. Thus, the importance of capital accumulation and the profit motive in the perpetuation of the HIV/AIDS crisis is ignored, or at least overshadowed.

Schulman's broad use of the term 'community' here also belies the rich and nuanced account of AIDS activism's textured (and often fraught) histories presented in the rest of *Let the Record Show*. She meticulously examines how society's broader power structures and material inequities were sometimes reproduced within activist circles, shining a light on some of the splinter groups that orbited larger AIDS organizations and advocated for HIV-positive women, people of color, and homeless or incarcerated individuals. Such groups experienced HIV/AIDS in different ways to the white gay men who largely represented the faces of AIDS activism. Women with AIDS, for example, often presented with different symptoms to men, such as irregular cervical smears or pelvic inflammatory disease. Meanwhile, the medical establishment refused to include women in medical research or pharmaceutical trials, largely due to a reluctance within this male-dominated sector to countenance what were considered fringe concerns that could ultimately be filed away as 'women's issues'. As a result, female HIV-positive activists

> died far more rapidly than some of the men. The reasons were socio-economic, and lack of access to health care. A lot of these women were way sicker than the men before seeking treatment, and they were not diagnosed until it was essentially too late. Many then had an aversion to swallowing the early medications because they hadn't been tested on women, and they didn't know what the dose would be, and it made them sick. (Schulman 2021a, 263)

Women PWAs also had to contend with neglect and dismissal from activist groups themselves. For example, for all the good he contributed to activist movements, Schulman claims, Larry Kramer failed to integrate the politics of women and people of color into his worldview. His laser focus on attracting the attention of powerful institutions meant Kramer uncritically exploited his own class privileges as a screenwriter and film producer to access media platforms and disseminate information about how AIDS was affecting gay male communities (Schulman 2021a, 175). To this end, he often avoided questions about how such institutional power dynamics operated. When exhorted by Schulman to refer reporters to women and people of color in ACT UP, for example, he tellingly responded: 'But Sarah, shouldn't we use our best people?' (qtd. in Schulman 2021a, 17). Sidelined in this way, HIV-positive individuals who did not fit the media's conceptualization of the PWA were incentivized to start thinking collectively and establish groups such as the National Women's Committee.

This splintering of AIDS activist groups stemmed, at least in part, from the material bases on which dominant hegemony rested. As historian Jonathan Bell notes, there were plenty of missteps taken on the part of groups like GMHC, which suffered from a certain class myopia at times. Take, for example, the ways in which the group poured their time and resources into supporting PWAs who attempted to take legal action against their employers for restricting healthcare access. While this move represented a pragmatic approach on a case-by-case basis, structurally it 'privileged those who actually had insurance already, and further consolidated the symbiotic relationship between the gay rights movement and private employment as the vehicle of social citizenship' (Bell 2018, 177). Thus, the crisis was 'degayed' to some extent, as activists and liberal Democrats 'openly embraced for sexual minorities a medical model that lifted them above the stigma of a public welfare system and integrated them further into heteronormative capitalism' (Bell 2018, 165). It should come as no surprise, perhaps, that efforts to counter this parochial politics were led most often by those on the peripheries – women and people of color whose lives depended on activism better attuned to the structural inequities and overlapping injustices that influenced how different constituencies experienced the HIV/AIDS crisis.

Thus, the countervailing interests that rippled through AIDS advocacy and activist groups in the 1980s and 1990s generated a fertile arena in which to exercise Bechtel's praxis of plurality and engage in the kind of dialectical struggle Kushner's play foregrounds. This is not, of course, to say that *Angels* presented a direct critique of ongoing strategies within AIDS activist movements. Rather, its willingness to consider the machinations of the socio-economic foundation from which seemingly unrelated inequities are borne might be instructive for political organizing across recent conjunctures. To see how this dissident spirit has emerged in practice, take the reaction to Marianne Elliott's 2017 production at London's National Theatre as an illustrative example. In the press, an overwhelming majority of critics highlighted the stark contemporaneity of *Angels*, pointing out the play's eerie resonance with a present characterized by Trumpian politics and runaway neoliberal capitalism. One, for example, emphasized Kushner's ability to tackle

> the shocking tardiness of the Reagan administration to respond to this crisis. And in some ways it is the political terrain of the play that hits most forcefully today. A scene in which Justice Department officials celebrate "the end of liberalism" has a chilling resonance, not least when you learn that Roy Cohn, the vicious, hypocritical lawyer who represents that mind-set here (and who denied his own sexuality and his affliction with Aids) was Trump's legal adviser for years. The portrait of a fractured America feels no less resonant today. (Hemming 2017)

Staged just after the inauguration of Donald Trump in 2017, those involved in this revival worked hard to emphasize the play's contemporaneous political resonances. The production program, for example, contains a full six pages dedicated to an article about the history of

Roy Cohn and his long association with Trump. As its writer Harry Scoble notes, 'It is unsettling to think that in fact the era of Roy Cohn's greatest political influence may have just begun' (National Theatre 2017, 44). By discussing topics as far-reaching and era-defining as the dissolution of the Soviet Union, climate change, and race relations against the backdrop of the AIDS crisis in America, *Angels* demands that we draw connections with past and ongoing political issues in this way. Casting the epidemic as a single node enmeshed in a larger network of interconnected issues, the play allows us to dodge at least some of the trappings of AIDS nostalgia on the contemporary stage.

To conclude this chapter, I want to clarify that *Angels* by no means represents the perfect counterhegemonic play or even a straightforwardly socialistic work. Rather, its playful contradictions, theoretical scaffolding, and cautiously revolutionary spirit are exceptional within what we might consider the mainstream of HIV/AIDS theater, thus laying the groundwork for a Gramscian critique of the genre and its historical development. Nor do I want to imply that the history of HIV/AIDS theater lacks radical voices or counterhegemonic work. The 1990s in particular witnessed a wave of so-called 'second-generational' HIV/AIDS plays that openly challenged neoliberal governance and conducted formal theatrical experiments toward political ends. Unlike *Angels*, however, these plays typically ignored how the pandemic compounded the subjugation and neglect of racialized people and women. In the absence of a Gramscian strategic consciousness, such plays offered a particularistic counterhegemony that was outspokenly gay and fearlessly experimental, but lacked the more universalist, dialectical politics necessary to comprehend and tackle the imbrications of race, class, stigma, and inequality in America. In the next chapter, therefore, before we explore how neoliberalism has affected HIV/AIDS theater after the millennium, we will consider the extent to which second-generational theater altered public consciousness surrounding HIV/AIDS.

CHAPTER TWO

Second-generation HIV/AIDS Theater

Around the mid-1990s, the HIV/AIDS theater genre started changing shape. Seemingly disillusioned with the earnest, educative work exemplified by Larry Kramer and William Hoffman, playwrights and directors started to create much more experimental and anti-assimilatory theater about the ongoing crisis.[1] Scholar Therese Jones termed this dissident body of work 'second-generation' theater, a temporal designation popularized by her edited anthology of American HIV/AIDS plays, *Sharing the Delirium: Second Generation AIDS Plays and Performances* (1994). As she explained in a publicity interview for the collection, 'First-generation plays like *As Is* and *The Normal Heart* were more traditional in form and definitely more sentimental [...] They were educationally driven. They disseminated information about AIDS to the gay community, as well as to the straight community about gays' (qtd. in Breslauer 1994). Second-generation plays, on the other hand, were much less focused on disseminating information designed to help individuals cope with the consequences of AIDS than they were on examining the wider political dimensions of the disease. This move away from health-oriented pedagogy liberated the genre to

1 While I do not examine Hoffman's *As Is* (1985) at any length in this study, it is worth noting its status as a piece of pioneering pedagogical work. As Astrid Haas explains, the play provided 'basic biomedical information about the syndrome in a factual yet gay- and sexuality-supportive manner far removed from the hysterical media coverage and devoid of the contradictions that characterized the discourse among medical scientists' (Haas 2011, 79). In so doing, it worked alongside Kramer's play to demystify the pandemic for a liberal theatergoing public.

a certain extent, allowing playwrights to produce work that was far more experimental in form and overtly political, resisting the urge to employ AIDS as 'a mechanism for humanizing or redeeming the gay character' (Jones qtd. in Breslauer 1994).

Dissatisfied with the assimilatory imperatives that appeared to burden their first-generational counterparts, then, second-generation playwrights were more than willing to criticize and ironize aspects of the dominant culture. Take Wendell Jones and David Stanley's *AIDS! The Musical!* (1991), for example – a deeply countercultural play featuring sex clubs, Radical Faeries, and new age gatherings in which characters describe their wishes to shoot George H. W. Bush and sing songs with refrains such as 'Momma, I need a gun for my birthday' (Jones and Stanley 1994, 230). Or take, instead, Doug Holsclaw's farce *The Baddest of Boys* (1992) – an acerbically black comedy which sees dying café owner Perry and his colleagues plan (or, in Perry's case, hallucinate) how to put him out of his misery using a range of brutal tools, including microwave radiation, a shotgun, a blowtorch, or carbon monoxide. Indeed, gallows humor and violent fantasies involving high-profile Republicans were common tropes threaded throughout second-generation theater – shock tactics designed to highlight the fatal neglect of US governance and initiate audience members into a community affectively connected by loss and oppression. This chapter examines the political valences of such counterhegemonic work to understand how playwrights combated rightward, homophobic tendencies during what could be described as the heyday of neoliberalism.

First, we will focus on how second-generation playwrights fought back against the millenarian tendencies that shaped American politics before the turn of the twenty-first century. From the apocalypticism of the Christian Right (who viewed AIDS as divine retribution for liberalism's sins) to the utopian millenarianism of neoliberal ideologues (who celebrated capitalism's apparent victory over socialist alternatives following the collapse of the Soviet Union), second-generation playwrights parodied conservative America's often-contradictory attachment to both extreme individualism and religious moral asceticism, with a view to building queer solidarity in the face of deep systemic oppression. Then, we will attend to the blind spots of second-generation work, vulnerable as it was to the individualist injunctions it ridiculed. As we will see, some of the genre's most audacious dissidents lacked the universalist consciousness necessary for understanding HIV/AIDS as a crisis extending far beyond the realms of white, gay, middle-class America. In constructing a particularistic politics of 'community' or 'alternative kinship' within bourgeois cultural institutions, many second-generation theater makers were oblivious to the ways in which historically dispossessed constituencies were locked out of such bounded structures. In turn, the experiences of HIV-positive people of color, women, and working-class people were almost entirely overlooked in second-generational theater. Finally, we will attend to one of the major exceptions to this exclusionary trend – Iranian-American avant-gardist Reza Abdoh, whose horror-inflected work attempted to raise consciousness about the effects of HIV/AIDS on the racialized and dispossessed by assaulting its audiences with scenes of intense violence and cruelty. Despite enjoying relative success when premiered (albeit wrapped in a healthy dose of scandal), Abdoh's work has received less critical examination within the field of HIV/AIDS theater scholarship compared to some of the more formally conventional plays cited in this book. To address this gap, we will consider the extent to which Abdoh's plays attacked naturalized neoliberal orthodoxies and how such orthodoxies might have affected the legacy of his work within the broader context of HIV/AIDS theater.

The radicality of second-generation HIV/AIDS theater

In the late 1990s and early noughties, the generational designation Jones set out in her edited anthology was generally well received among queer scholars and theater practitioners. With queer theory emerging as an influential field of critical studies, art that subverted societal norms or 'heteronormativity' through experimentation was seen to reflect this radical scholarly turn. Writing in 2001, for example, Torsten Graff asserted:

> Over the last decade, gay drama has become more and more queer. The subtitle of Therese Jones's anthology [...] indicates not only a changed political, social and medical context for AIDS plays and performances, but simultaneously highlights a shift in the dramatic representation of AIDS. While the AIDS plays of the eighties were highly conventional plays in the tradition of naturalism and realism, dramatic texts of the past ten years [...] cannot be adequately understood without queer theory or the influence of more than a decade of queer ACT-UP activism. (Graff 2001, 23)

Understanding this link between theory, action, and queer realpolitik is vital for examining the development of second-generation theater.

Having captured the attention of the American public and, to a lesser extent, other publics in the Global North via widely dispersed chapters, ACT UP steered the queer counterattack against oppressive governance and engaged in a kind of Gramscian war of position – stealthy and gradual engagement in cultural struggle as a means to build (counter)hegemonic support.

As Tamar W. Carroll explains, the group's memorable collective actions – which included successfully seizing control of the US Food and Drug Administration (FDA) in 1988 and enveloping the home of brazenly homophobic US Senator Jesse Helms in a giant, 15-foot condom in 1991 – were examples of the group's engagement with the so-called 'culture wars' that were taking place in the US at the time. Often used as a catch-all term to describe the antagonisms felt between conservative ideologues and progressive voices across a range of social justice movements, the culture wars were 'directly tied to the Religious Right and pro-family movement's attempts to regulate national morality and to conservatives' successful attacks on the welfare state' (Carroll 2015, 136). Interested in preserving the private realm of the family unit, religious conservatives viewed abortion and gay rights as overstretching the function of the state. As such, evangelicals and other religious conservatives joined forces with neoliberal conservatives in their efforts to slash social welfare programs. This neoconservative–neoliberal coalition, an often paradoxical relationship this chapter will explore in detail, deployed the rhetoric of (economic) freedom to shore up consent for policies that further impoverished the marginalized, restricting bodily autonomy and demonizing those who refused to conform to normative familial structures. Such a hostile climate galvanized the anti-establishment fervor of second-generational playwrights and helped to shape the new, 'queerer' dramatic representations of AIDS that Graff observes.

So, queerness as an explicatory and political framework had the potential to tackle and subvert at least some of neoliberalism's cruelest oppressive imperatives. It is worth noting at this point, of course, that the term 'queer' is wildly polysemic, etymologically complex, and always vulnerable to misinterpretation when deployed in a scholarly context. As Peter Drucker notes, 'no single word – neither "queer" nor any other – can fully encompass the broad discourse that is needed by the LGBT left' (Drucker 2015, 11). This is reflected by queer's inability to elude co-optation by the dominant culture, as seen, for example, in the popularity of reality television shows such as *Queer Eye*, which conceptualizes queerness as a kind of key to self-betterment within the competitive dominant hegemony (Sackur 2019). In the context of this study, then, I use 'queer' as shorthand to describe a spirit of anti-normativity and anti-identitarianism, placing particular emphasis on its utility in anti-capitalist discourse. Queerness – in opposition to gay consumer culture and assimilation into heterosexual kinship paradigms – 'still implies, as it has done since its emergence as a current in the early 1990s, rebellion and gender bending' (Drucker 2015, 11). In so doing, queer subcultures challenge neoliberal capitalism's fetishization of productivism, which inculcates in people the urgency of economic growth and, by extension, exhorts them to climb career ladders, purchase property, and (for women) procreate before their 'biological clocks' run over.

Such 'milestones' appeared arbitrary and limiting to the queer vanguard of the 1990s. Leo Bersani, for example, analyzed the hegemonic foundations on which America's obsession with familial longevity and lineage was built in his polemical *Homos* (1995), ultimately demanding for queer communities 'a future without discrimination even as AIDS makes us wonder how much of a future we have' (Bersani [1995] 2009, 20). Relatedly, second-generation playwrights also cast aside future-oriented heteronormativity in favor of a politics of the present, trivializing and satirizing hegemonic narratives surrounding familial duty. As Noreen Barnes-McLain noted, HIV/AIDS plays of the mid-1990s were concerned with 'the *quality* of time spent while living. As in the first wave of works, there is no question of whether one will die, and how one meets one's death is still the central action of the play' (Barnes-McLain 1997, 117).

The rift between dominant attitudes toward (productive) temporality and a life well lived, and those of queer artists and scholars, took on heightened dimensions in the American culture wars of the late twentieth century. As the year 2000 approached, millenarianism – the politically or religiously motivated belief in imminent and groundbreaking societal transformation – gathered momentum. For the country's neoconservative Christian Right, AIDS represented a plague sent by God to punish those engaged in non-normative sex and secure America's future as a (re)productivist and imperialist state. The cultural fiction that the AIDS crisis represented an apocalyptic reckoning for queer or dissident communities is analyzed at length in Thomas L. Long's *AIDS and American Apocalypticism: The Cultural Semiotics of an Epidemic* (2005). Long observes that political action groups such as the 'Moral Majority' and television evangelists like Pat Robertson and Jerry Falwell 'had already constructed homosexuality itself as a contagious disease and as an apocalyptic signifier' by the late 1970s (Long 2005, 2). The emergence of AIDS, therefore, appeared to corroborate their discriminatory diagnosis. Although such venomous sentiment was largely contained within parochial evangelical groups, millenarian rhetoric seeped into wider governmental and social realms by promoting neoconservative moralism in a way that fortified some of the profoundly Americentric and individualistic rationalities endorsed by neoliberal hegemony.

It would be difficult to overstate the political might of the neoconservative–neoliberal coalition that queer constituencies and people with HIV found themselves up against in the US. When the AIDS crisis took hold, homonormativity had not shored up the (admittedly precarious) hegemonic influence it enjoys today, so the broadcast of emphatically homophobic sentiment by evangelicals was relatively permissible within wider society. Heterosexual coupling and nuclear familial relations were endorsed in a way that sated neoconservative beliefs in regulatory moralism while simultaneously feeding neoliberal imperatives surrounding unbridled economic growth, with the traditional family unit conceptualized as a fertile unit within which to exploit labor and accumulate capital. At first glance, this consonance of ideologies might appear unlikely – neoconservatism's various attachments to family and religious values, isolationism, and material asceticism seem to directly oppose neoliberalism's ostensible *raison d'être* – financial growth bolstered by hyper-individualist subjectivities. Political theorist Wendy Brown has offered some of the most lucid and comprehensive accounts of this durable and distinctly American alliance. In the mid-2000s, Brown took stock of the ongoing negotiation between neoconservatism and neoliberalism in her essay 'American Nightmare: Neoliberalism, Neoconservatism, and De-Democratization' (2006). Although neoliberalism's tendency to propagate the wealth of the already-rich runs counter to neoconservatism's reliance on working-class support and the valorization of a (nuclear) family wage, she argued, state powers resolved this tension through the hegemonization of wealth as inherently 'American'. The country's imperial power on the world stage became an element of patriotic attachment, rendering 'anti-American any resentment of the rich' and rationalizing a deteriorating standard of existence for working-class constituencies (Brown 2006, 701).

More recently, Brown has refined this thesis in the wake of Trumpism. The emergence of increasingly authoritarian and socially conservative imperatives among the American political class, she argues, can be traced back to key principles held by neoliberalism's earliest scholarly architects. For Friedrich Hayek, for example, 'the relation of markets and morals in the neoliberal project has nothing to do with supplements, hybridity, resonance, convergence, or mutual exploitation. Rather, markets and morals, equally important to a thriving civilization, are rooted in a common ontology of spontaneously evolved orders borne by tradition' (Brown 2019, 96). The free and creative capacity to shape society, Hayek believed, emerged organically from below. As such, he viewed the version of freedom ascribed to the social democratic state as delusional and as laying the groundwork for totalitarianism. While neoliberalism's hegemonic project is undoubtedly elastic enough to subsume a variety of viewpoints that dispute such claims, Hayek's faith in human beings' essential tendency toward private property, gender conformity, and social atomism goes some way toward elucidating why the most reactionary echelons of right-wing America have been so invested in neoliberal capitalism from the 1980s to the present day.

Given the systematic oppression and degradation many second-generation playwrights experienced as a result of this neoconservative–neoliberal alliance, they were highly attuned to its machinations. Take Paul Rudnick's *The Most Fabulous Story Ever Told* (1998), for example. Having gained commercial success both on and off Broadway for his camply risqué and sharply insightful comedies, Rudnick was well placed to satirize the dangerous alliance between conservative religiosity and neoliberal capitalism at the turn of the millennium. *Fabulous* reimagines the story of Genesis and other fragments of the Old Testament to achieve this aim. Gay lovers Adam and Steve fill in for the traditional Adam and Eve, subverting the tired conservative slogan 'God made Adam and Eve, not Adam and Steve', while lesbian couple Jane and Mabel make for somewhat less direct spin-offs of Cain and Abel. Building on this spirit of parody and biblical subversion, the four characters spend the beginning of the play's first act negotiating friendship, sex, wealth, divinity, and even bestiality in a world with no former civilization to guide them, with the act closing just before Jesus' birth.

The second act is set in modern-day New York on Christmas Eve. Both couples are still together but remember nothing of their biblical selves. On top of this, Steve is infected with HIV and Jane has become pregnant via artificial insemination. Such a set-up invites comparisons between the biblical and modern-day versions of the characters, and by extension the ways in which religion continues to have a bearing on modern-day neoliberal America. As William E. Burns explains, some variants of Christian millenarian doctrine, which anticipate 1,000 years of perfect life on Earth before the Last Judgment, posit that the society that exists during such a millennium 'would be perfect, with total human command over nature paralleling the command over nature that Adam had enjoyed in the Garden of Eden before the Fall' (Burns 2011, 198). The first half of *Fabulous*, then, can be analyzed as a millenarian text in terms of its portrayal of Eden, its providential tone, and its brand of future-oriented theological discussion. The play's second half then goes on to deconstruct religious chiliasm and its secular parallels by asking questions about the legacy of HIV/AIDS, the future of the economy, and its fraught yet tight-knit relationship with Christianity in contemporary America.

Despite Rudnick's obvious desire to undermine homophobic apocalypticism, *Fabulous* refuses to present the problem as an epiphenomenal pathology of right-wing ideology. From the outset, Rudnick uses dialectical techniques to untangle how wider hegemonic forces have contributed to the systematic oppression of the queer and HIV-positive, taking light-hearted aim at a variety of religious and political viewpoints and emphasizing their mutually reinforcing roles in upholding hegemonic standards. In so doing, he parodies the development of what Jason Hackworth describes as 'religious neoliberalism'. For Hackworth, one cannot explain neoliberalism's ideational rise through economic concepts and state rationalities alone. Viewing its hegemonic power as intertwined with (neo-)Calvinist philosophies that elevate the moral value of work, he argues, can help explain why neoliberalism 'is so appealing during times of crisis when it has such a clear track record of long- and medium-term failure' (Hackworth 2012, 12). More specifically, religious neoliberalism explains why America's neoconservatives are often so attached to 'prosperity theology', a concept promoting the idea that God rewards faithful followers with material wealth. As Hackworth notes, a 'variety of biblical verses are used to justify the position that God wants his followers to be prosperous' (Hackworth 2012, 41), such as the following from Deuteronomy: 'You must remember the LORD your God, for he is the one who gives ability to get wealth; if you do this he will confirm his covenant that he made by oath to your ancestors, even as he has to this day' (Deut. 8:18). The idea that God rewards faithful followers with material wealth reinforces Calvinist tenets of individual responsibility for one's success and failures. Furthermore, it justifies the neoliberal imperative to dissolve the welfare state and 'sanctifies property as an expression of piety' (Hackworth 2012, 45).

Parodic examples of prosperity theology start to appear in *Fabulous* after the Fall. Having, in Steve's words, built a 'casual and elegant lifestyle' for themselves, the group list the wonders of a range of their inventions from the wheel to two-in-one shampoo and conditioner.

Adam then pulls out a Bible, exclaiming 'as of today, we have all been together for 400 years. And I think we look great!' (Rudnick 2010, 167). He then opines, 'And yet – our happiness hasn't been complete. We have each other, we have so much, but still – we know nothing. We have no answers. Until – right now!', going on to introduce the group to the idea of God (Rudnick 2010, 167). In line with the notion of prosperity theology, reaching 'completion' would necessitate a reward that transcends any of the material comforts they have previously experienced. Although the trajectory of Rudnick's version of Genesis diverges greatly from the biblical version – not least due to the non-generative potential of the protagonists' same-sex relationships – I conjecture that Adam's decision to mark the 400th year of their postlapsarian existence could represent a loose reference to the following verse in Genesis: 'Then the LORD said to Abram, "Know for certain that your descendants will be strangers in a foreign country. They will be enslaved and oppressed for four hundred years. But I will execute judgement on the nation that they will serve. Afterward they will come out with many possessions' (Gen. 15:13–14). Clearly, this promise of material reward for serving God for 400 years might be interpreted as exemplary of prosperity theology, exciting a kind of millenarian consciousness that looks forward to revelatory reward after centuries of suffering. In adopting this rather obscure reference to vaunt the individual success and attractiveness of his peers, Adam parodies contemporary hegemony's figuring of 'citizens as individual entrepreneurs and consumers whose moral autonomy is measured by their capacity for "self-care"' (Brown 2006, 694), while revealing the shared ideological imperatives between religious millenarianism and (at least ostensibly) secular neoliberalism.

As neoliberal regimes hailed the dawn of a revolutionary new capitalism, quasi-religious hope surrounding economic stability emerged. As noted in a premillennial issue of the socialist magazine *Monthly Review*,

> A dynamic global economy that has no precedents is said to be propelling the world into a new millennium of abundance. In their 1998 special double issue on 'The 21st Century Economy', for instance, the editors of Business Week predicted that "Revolutionary technology and rapid globalization [...] will send productivity soaring, allowing faster growth with low inflation and modest unemployment". This dynamic would last for decades, bringing unimagined prosperity worldwide. (McNally 1999)

It is the 'unimagined' element of such prosperity that renders this mode of thinking millenarian and represents a school of thought popularized by key neoliberal proponents during the late twentieth century. In 1989, for example, Francis Fukuyama, galvanized by the ongoing collapse of the Soviet Union and a brief stint of strong economic growth across much of the Western world, prophesied the long-term triumph of economic liberalism in a now-infamous essay, 'The End of History?'. For Fukuyama, the end of the Cold War and the seeming triumph over fascism and communism across much of the world reflected 'the total exhaustion of viable systematic alternatives to Western liberalism', a conclusion he claimed to have reached via Hegelian dialectical theory (Fukuyama 1989, 3). The theoretical framework on which Fukuyama hangs his essay vehemently rejects the materialist dialectics associated with Marxist thought, which he blames for almost occasioning nuclear war. Vowing to 'save' Hegel's philosophy from its associations with Marx, whose works were inspired by Hegelian dialectics, he argues for an idealist conceptualization of consciousness as potentially autonomous from the development of the material world and at the same time capable of effecting change within it.

The Marxist tradition, meanwhile, Fukuyama argues, relegates 'the entire realm of consciousness – religion, art, culture, philosophy itself – to a "superstructure" that was determined entirely by the prevailing material mode of production' (Fukuyama 1989, 6). Of course, this is despite the fact that Marxist thinkers had been troubling and reevaluating the base–superstructure framework for years by the time this essay was published, demonstrating how Fukuyama slicks an expedient gloss over certain forms of leftist scholarship to support his notion that the modern liberal state has secured humanity's right to freedom and democracy through 'ideological evolution' (Fukuyama 1989, 4). Although Western liberal democracy had not, Fukuyama claimed, yet asserted itself in many developing nations, he cites the adoption of essentially neoliberal structures in China under Deng Xiao-Ping as evidence that the ideology was working its way through an increasingly globalized world, destined to become 'the end point of mankind's evolution and [...] the final form of human government' (Fukuyama 1989, 4). With democratic freedoms secured and ideological conflicts consigned to the past, Fukuyama's theoretical homogeneous world free of history could be left to run primarily on economic activity and the willingness of self-disciplining subjects to serve the interests of capital, thus minimizing the need for state governance.

To today's readers, it is probably fairly obvious why Fukuyama's ideas have been progressively more reviled as global political ruptures have continued to unfold over the third millennium. From the election of aspiring autocrats to the escalation of ecological crises, the evidence against the 'end of history' thesis is stacking up. Such a vantage point allows us to vindicate Rudnick's critique of neoliberalism and its contribution to the suffering of the queer and HIV-positive. Toward the end of *Fabulous,* discussion of Steve's HIV/AIDS serves as a kind of epilogue, exposing the ways in which, despite its seemingly greater acceptance of gay people, contemporary neoliberal–neoconservative America continues to punish non-normative sexualities. Attentive audience members watching Act Two should be able to recall that Steve sets out for Sodom in the first act of the play, saying of Adam, 'I don't want him back! I want a new boyfriend! No, I want lots of new boyfriends! A new one every night, every minute! I'm sick of being in love! Where can I go? To meet every man who isn't Adam?' (Rudnick 2010, 196). Steve's HIV, which is eventually revealed to be drug-resistant, can therefore be read as viral retribution for his transgressive desires; even in a liberal world where homosexuality is permissible, non-monogamy remains an immoral and punishable act.

The use of the sodomitic trope to punish not gay male sex but non-monogamy therefore appears as a parodic criticism of popular gay commentators such as Larry Kramer, who, at least in some respects, proffered socially conservative opinions. In a screed against the kind of casual sex Steve searches for in *Fabulous,* Kramer states, 'You cannot fuck indiscriminately with multiple partners, who are also doing the same, without spreading disease, a disease that has for many years also carried death. Nature always extracts a price for sexual promiscuity' (Kramer 1997). By bestowing such agency upon nature and rendering it god-like, Kramer employs a logic akin to that of prosperity theology, demonstrating how seemingly secular arguments can emulate and corroborate the puritanical doctrine of the Religious Right. As Eric Rofes has observed, the rhetoric of queer commentators such as Kramer or John Rechy 'often default[s] to solutions to complex social problems that are uncannily similar to strategies embraced by neoconservative social critics' (Rofes 1998, 159). Rudnick's evocation of Sodom, then, in its subversive appropriation, can be read as a means to expose the specious reasoning behind the chiliastic/apocalyptic rhetoric espoused even by queer-identified groups toward the end of the twentieth century.

The interrogation of millenarian and religious attitudes toward HIV/AIDS becomes increasingly explicit as *Fabulous* reaches its conclusion. Although Steve seroconverts after the introduction of life-saving protease inhibitors (or as Mabel calls the 28 pills he has to ingest a day, 'twenty-eight miracles'), Rudnick shuts down any temptation to interpret this good fortune as evidence of divine intervention: in the play's closing lines, Steve reveals that his HIV is drug-resistant (Rudnick 2010, 230). He tells Adam, 'Look, they don't work for everyone, and no one's been on them that long, and the side effects are worse than the disease' (Rudnick 2010, 241). Here, Rudnick highlights the arbitrary and capricious nature of disease, and the error in trying to make sense of it purely through the lens of religion or theology. The corollary to this is his subsequent renunciation of other secular forms of millenarianism. For example, when Steve's predicament ultimately causes Adam to renounce his faith in God, he finds immediate comfort in the Christmas present Steve gives him, excitedly proclaiming, 'Oh my God. You got it. This is just what I wanted. This is cashmere. This is Armani. This cost a fortune' (Rudnick 2010, 242). In so easily casting off his faith in favor of consumerism and wealth, Adam reveals certain aspects of religion and neoliberal consumerism to be interchangeable, illuminating the similarities that lie at their heart. I therefore detect a kind of Gramscian consciousness in *Fabulous* that views religiosity as bound up with corollary secular norms. As Gramsci specifies in the *Notebooks*, 'religion is an element of fragmented common sense' that colludes with other ideas from the realms of ideology, folklore, and superstition to generate ideas that appear natural, eternal, and immune to change (Gramsci 2003, 325). In fact, '[t]he principal elements of common sense are provided by religion, and consequently the relationship between common sense and religion is much more intimate than that between common sense and the philosophical systems of the intellectuals' (Gramsci 2003, 420).

Another cultural producer keen to undermine the common-sense rationalisms that converged to generate this distinctly millennial phenomenon was solo performer Tim Miller, who vociferously attacked AIDS apocalypticism in a work titled *My Queer Body*. Hailed by Long as a 'queer evangelist', Miller employed the millenarian grammar of Christian evangelical oratory tradition to denounce neoliberal culture, taking on the role of (in his words) 'a sweaty tent-revival preacher' (Miller 2002, xviii). During the performance, Miller ruminates on the seemingly apocalyptic nature of AIDS before disseminating a chiliastic entreaty for queer liberation and utopianism in the upcoming millennium. Long notes that 'Miller has been variously compared to an evangelist, a preacher, and a pastor', appropriating a brand of rhetoric and audience participation in his performance pieces stylistically akin to that of Jerry Falwell or Pat Robertson (Long 2005, 38). However, in diametric opposition to the evangelists of this homophobic ilk, the focus of Miller's work is almost exclusively the subject of his own queerness; providing an autobiographical history of his body and the ways in which it can 'shine a light on systems of prejudice that are just so damn unfair' (Miller 2002, xvi).

Unlike *Fabulous*, which was (perhaps unexpectedly) embraced by the mainstream theatergoing establishment and helped secure Rudnick's reputation as a talented name on Broadway, Miller's work was subsumed by the culture wars and held up as exemplary of society's moral degradation by US conservatives. Initially pegged for a grant backed by the US National Endowment for the Arts (NEA), Miller's work was derided as 'indecent' by NEA chairman John Frohnmeyer and all funding was vetoed under the aegis of a so-called 'decency clause', along with that of three other performance artists – Karen Finley, Holly Hughes, and John Fleck. Known as the 'NEA Four', the group were united by their willingness to explore themes of sexuality, gender, and the trauma of living outside of America's rigid heteronorm. Although the group successfully won a district court battle against the government following the controversy, the Supreme Court ruled in 1998 that the clause did not disrupt artists' First Amendment rights. Following pressure from an increasingly rightward government, the NEA stopped funding individual artists altogether – a rule that persists to this day.

Stigmatized as an objectionable figure in the public consciousness, Miller had to perform *MQB* in small student-run theaters and queer venues, meaning its appeal was largely confined to a limited cohort of gay men. As one student reviewer noted of an early performance of *MQB*, 'the audience, primarily composed of gay male couples, filtered in. There was a certain sense of isolation involved in being in the midst of a group where everyone knew everyone else, and greetings between them flew thick and fast' (Sukthankar 1992). Miller was under no illusion as to the relatively niche nature of his work, of course, and exploited his outsider status to galvanize counterhegemonic fervor in the auditorium. In a much-cited essay co-authored with David Román, 'Preaching to the Converted', Miller makes a claim for the political importance of such queer gatherings, noting that, historically, queer theater has offered much political value to marginalized groups. While forging new communities might seem politically limited in the context of late capitalism, building groups of people with similar interests and coherent priorities is vital for any counterhegemonic project, equipping participants with the mental stamina and rhetorical tools they need to attract more people to their cause. As such, the 'history of lesbian and gay theatre accepts the notion of community as axiomatic and stages the struggle to sustain and expand community as one of its primary objectives' (Miller and Román 1995, 173–4). In this way, Miller's work was not developed with the aim of appealing to or addressing mainstream audiences, seeking instead to assist the already-marginalized in developing visions for a brighter future free from oppression.

One of the best examples of Miller's counterhegemonic (and humorous) approach appears at the beginning of *MQB*, when he imagines his own genesis as a 'queer little spermlet':

> A hideous sperm that looks like Jesse Helms tries to catch me in a net. I elude him! A herd of sperm who look like the military Joint Chiefs of Staff try to kick me out of this fallopian tube! I elude them, as well. Then a bunch of hulking macho slimebag straight-pig sperm shove and try to elbow me out of the way... And... ECCE HOMO!!! Behold the fag. And the big cry to the universe. Time to be born. (Miller 1994, 312)

'Ecce homo' – translated as 'behold the man' from the Vulgate version of John 19:5 – is the phrase used by Pontius Pilate when he presents Jesus Christ to the crowd awaiting his crucifixion. In equating his newborn self with a scourged Christ, Miller assumes a pedagogical role; an exilic prophet for the queer and marginalized. By evoking the figure of Senator Jesse Helms as a primary adversary, Miller embraces wholesale his own implication in the culture wars. As mentioned earlier in this chapter, Helms was a target for ACT UP's direct actions, due in large part to his role in introducing a series of congressional amendments that prevented federal funds 'from being used to provide AIDS education, information, or prevention materials and activities that promote, encourage, and condone homosexual sexual activities' (Helms 1987). In addition, he was directly involved in NEA censorship and, consistent with the neoliberal drive for privatization, wanted all public arts funding to be abolished. That Miller invokes Helms in the form of a 'hideous sperm', at its most patent level, illustrates Miller's opposition to these politics. Furthermore, by using the language of reproduction and gynecology, Miller invokes questions surrounding inherence and innateness. He playfully questions whether Jesse Helms was destined to oppress his art and that of his contemporaries due to some kind of genetic default, or whether he has fallen prey to robust hegemonic forces that have the potential to be denaturalized.

The first half of *MQB* answers these questions in an apocalyptic and fatalistic fashion, recounting scenes of queer death and destruction from the scourge of AIDS. Miller describes the 'volcano' of his life, inhabiting a 'City of plague. Government of hate' (Miller 1994,

322), going on to describe how 'Blood pours from here and here where the catheters pierced my friends' sides so the medicine could go in their bodies. AIDS! AIDS! Broken here where Reagan and Bush smiled their do-nothing holocaust grins while my friends died' (Miller 1994, 325), the incendiary evocation of past atrocity serving to compound his opposition to the neoliberal governance of these presidents. That the 'do-nothing' quality of their grins could lead to such atrocity is a damning indictment of an anti-interventionist state that places the responsibility for the economic stability, health, and wellbeing of its citizens largely on the citizens themselves. However, as Long notes, 'Although employing apocalyptic tropes – beasts, catastrophe, defilement, sacred eros – Miller was also repudiating the apocalyptic trajectory, first by climax's closure, then by rescripting the Western mythos of the Fall – the event upon which apocalyptic closure is predicated – by refusing to leave the Garden in the first place' (Long 2005, 44). Miller disrupts the chiliastic trope of AIDS apocalypticism utilized by orators on the Religious Right by realizing that – by virtue of his status as 'preacher' – he has power over the oration, and is able to relay his preferred vision of the future: 'Maybe I can make up a new ending and maybe we'll find our way out of the volcano' (Miller 1994, 328). It is at this point in the performance that Miller renounces apocalyptic millenarianism for its closely related utopian variant, telling his (largely queer) audiences, 'We're in a universe of our own making. No more waiting. Our hoped for escape from gravity. Weightless. We're in our own solar system' (Miller 1994, 334). Miller's encouragement to see beyond gravity or the solar system – phenomena whose existence scientific consensus tells us are immutable truths – acts as a metaphor for contemporary hegemony. He asks audiences to look beyond the common-sense orthodoxies pushed by neoliberalism in order to establish a pathway for queer liberation.

The limitations of queer politics in second-generation HIV/AIDS theater

Although second-generation plays employed an anti-capitalist tenor to galvanize their audiences, their adoption of a community-oriented queer politics was limited in its ability to critique the material bases upon which the oppression of HIV-positive people depends. Certainly, both Rudnick's and Miller's plays incisively critique the hubristic 'end of history' narrative espoused by their governments and neoliberal persecutors. However, their portrayal of the HIV/AIDS crisis as a kind of moral struggle and their reification of queer community as a circumscribed and straightforwardly intelligible instrument in the fight against oppression allowed them to overlook the contingent and relational nature of capitalism. In other words, while pointing out Jesse Helms' moral wrongs might whip up a communitarian political fervor, it focuses our attention primarily on the *effects* of an oppressive system, rather than its internal dynamics. As Rahel Jaeggi succinctly puts it, 'freestanding moral critique is never really able to pin the injustices it identifies *on capitalism*. Of course, capitalism was exploitative and unfair. But so was ancient slave society, and so was feudalism' (Fraser and Jaeggi 2018, 122).

In critiquing the effects of capitalism that specifically faced often white, often moneyed gay men populating US theaters in the early 1990s, therefore, second-generation playwrights overlooked the ways in which poor and racialized HIV-positive people encountered different challenges within the capitalist order. As Alberto Sandoval-Sánchez argues in a study exploring Latinos on and off Broadway, Therese Jones's conceptualization of second-generational gallows humor as politically subversive suffers, in some ways, from class myopia, noting that 'gay, white theater on AIDS [...] can afford to laugh in the 1990s; these people have learned how to cope and survive through camp and irony', without assessing the extent to which class has shaped their perspectives and philosophies (Sandoval-Sánchez 1999, 130). After all, it is easier to spend time laughing with friends when you are not confronted by additional worries such as surviving on a meager wage or covering healthcare costs. In highlighting the questionable class politics of second-generational theater, Sandoval-Sánchez hits upon wider critiques recently leveled against the queer politics and theory that informed HIV/AIDS activism and performance cultures in the US (and, to some extent, the UK and Canada).

Over the past decade or so, Marxist-oriented scholars including James Penney, Holly Lewis, and Christopher Chitty, among others, have started to challenge queer theoretical orthodoxies for their lack of materialist analysis and inadequate consideration of class struggle, particularly regarding the ability of poor and non-white people to come out and reject imperatives to adhere to familial expectations, raise children, etc. As Penney notes, vanguard texts that comprised the queer turn of the 1990s often relied on a voluntaristic politics incompatible with the exigencies of material survival for the working classes, thus tacitly or naively interpellating a higher-classed subject. Critiquing the psychoanalytic 'anti-relational' queer theory of Jack Halberstam and Lee Edelman, for example, he explains that 'queer discourse clings anxiously, if ironically, to the idea of an "us," apparently unable to let go of the notion despite the lack of convincing political or theoretical arguments in its favor' (Penney 2014, 13). Similarly for Chitty, the anti-identitarianism and 'anti-normativity' historically animating the notion of the queer tends unwittingly to fold in on itself as a form of liberationist politics. Adopting a Gramscian idiom, Chitty proffers an incisive reassessment of the emancipatory potential of queer identification in a world hostile to 'less productive' ways of living:

> Forms of love and life not limited to same-sex object choice but nonetheless "queer" correspond structurally to the historical position occupied by homosexuals, one outside the institutions of family, state, and couple form. As a social category, "queer" would then describe the morbid cultural forms by which the normative logics of gender and sexuality become irreparably damaged, desperately reasserted, and perversely renaturalized within a generalized social crisis – rather than marking some utopian release from these logics in the pursuit of self-transformative play. Against the background of widespread infrastructural fallout, the normal persists within decrepit forms, remaining in force but with significantly weakened powers. (Chitty 2020, 188)

To place faith in the queer as an immanently insubordinate force, then, is to ignore the ways in which subaltern groups' self-understanding is necessarily – ineluctably – generated by the sexual norms of the dominant hegemon. With this in mind, to what extent can organizing on the basis of a shared queer self-understanding tackle capitalism's material oppressions?

Miranda Joseph's *Against the Romance of Community* (2002) remains instructive when answering such a question. In her work, Joseph combines ethnographic research with Marxist theory to make the case that the contemporary notion of community as a coalition of interrelated individuals that lies outside of – or stands counter to – wider hegemonic structures is both idealistic and blind to the role that capitalism plays in shaping shared identities. In consonance with Chitty, she argues 'against the idea that communities are organic, natural, spontaneous occurrences', pointing out that constructing prosocial groups around a particular identity formation (and, therefore, implicitly *in opposition* to others) often represents an adaptive effort to *mitigate* capitalism's materially rapacious effects and psychic traumas, rather than address their root causes (Joseph 2002, viii). A queer community that creates a so-called 'chosen family' in response to rejection by biological kin, for example, might help its members survive capitalism's cruelties while simultaneously satisfying capital's need for unwaged socially reproductive labor. Lacking a universalistic political consciousness that identifies ostensibly social relations as really relations between things (following Marx's construction of fetishism), identitarianism cannot address the internal dynamics of capitalism; instead, it unwittingly ingeminates and rigidifies extant power structures. To put it another way, as John Holloway succinctly argues, the dialectical thought which remains so constructive in anti-capitalist critique is by its nature 'the "consistent sense of non-identity", the sense of the explosive force of that which is denied' (Holloway 2010, 76).

Attempts to redress material dispossession and related societal oppression via a realpolitik grounded in delimited community spirit, therefore, leave queer community vulnerable to cooptation and subversion by hegemonic forces. As Joseph explains, the discourse of community has been increasingly adopted to bolster corporate endeavors in an age of free-market fundamentalism, with communal subjectivity often constituted by the capitalist practices of production and consumption (Joseph 2002, viii). The more communities an individual (or consumer) is able to identify with, the greater the potential for corporate gain. The attempt to appeal to communitarian notions of multiculturalism and diversity has shifted from being a tool of nonprofits and educational institutions to one embraced by corporations, allowing them to subsume broad desires for sociality into exploitative capitalist practices: 'diversity discourse deploys existing differences and elaborates new ones as occasions for the voluntary and enthusiastic participation of subjects as niched or individuated producers and consumers' (Joseph 2002, 22). Within the institution of theater, which is by no means immune to corporatism, community-oriented projects aimed at particular so-called 'demographics' might reveal distinctly neoliberal imperatives.

I am not aiming to downplay the ways in which queer community theater shone a light on pressing political issues, fostered solidaristic ties, and offered genuine material and psychic benefits to subsections of HIV-positive people during the 1990s, when second-generation playwrights were primarily active. Rather, I invoke Joseph's work to trouble conceptualizations of the institution of theater as a 'natural' facilitator of communal relations, as well as representations of community as unequivocally 'good' or 'progressive'. To flesh out why such an analysis is vital to any materialist reading of HIV/AIDS theater, I turn to Joseph's in-depth ethnographic study of Theatre Rhinoceros, a nonprofit gay and lesbian theater company based in San Francisco that was founded in 1977 to provide LGBTQ-identifying performers with a platform for their work and to 'diversify' the city's theatrical offerings. Having spent time behind the scenes observing meetings involving the company's artistic directors and board members in the early 1990s, Joseph asserts that we should be suspicious of claims to diversity and inclusivity. She describes an atmosphere of so-called 'homosexism' in the meetings: a 'prioritization of gayness over other identity features' that saw company members subordinating the work of bisexual playwrights or, indeed, any plays that did not fit in to their ideal notions of (primarily white and male) gay theater (Joseph 2002, xvii). Noting that both artistic directors had actually assumed the job titles of gay men who had been struck down by AIDS, Joseph explains that,

> Adele [Prandini] and Doug [Holsclaw] gained a great deal of authority by inscribing themselves into the traumatic and oppressed history of the theatre and community. It was Doug's habitual role in staff meetings to recall and defend the way things had always been done. And throughout [one such] meeting, both Doug and Adele were able to represent the needs and desires of 'the community' in a way that trumped all other suggestions. (Joseph 2002, xiii)

As evidenced by Joseph's interviews with frequenters of the venue, conducted around 1991, 'the way things had always been done' pertained to the stories of relatively well-off white gay men living in San Francisco. While Prandini emphasized her supposed ambitions to include new and diverse voices in the theater's annual program, the stories of these men were seen as what its community desired, and therefore, presumably, the theater's primary income generators.

In order to intervene in what was clearly a hierarchy that privileged certain voices in the theater, its artistic directors set up an initiative to encourage 'diversity'. However, as Joseph explains, its success was very much reliant on rigidifying and strengthening the identitarian hierarchies against which it was supposedly pushing:

> The development project involved the linked political and economic goals of forging a multicultural gay community and creating work of quality (and cost) that would be equivalent to that found in mainstream theater. These goals were linked through a series of programs that were intended to do both things at once. But such "development" depended on contributions from the gay community, contributions from artists of their work, and contributions from audience members through their subscriptions and financial donations. Adele thus cast the development

> programs as themselves gifts to the community in relation to which the community should reciprocate. (Joseph 2002, 106)

Perhaps unsurprisingly, most of the audience members who had the financial means to contribute to the program were precisely 'those white gay men who had been the primary addressees of the theater's productions over the years' and whose continued representation onstage was essentially, therefore, secured through gift donations (Joseph 2002, 107).

Such philanthropic gifts are very much implicated in neoliberal ideology, despite their apparent generosity. In some ways, Theatre Rhinoceros's community funding initiative represents a small-scale version of what has come to be known as 'philanthrocapitalism' – a situation whereby wealthy individuals channel money toward charitable or prosocial causes they deem most worthy, determining how best to address societal problems without democratic input from beneficiaries or their wider community. Within the context of Theatre Rhinoceros's diversity program, wealthy donors were rewarded with the opportunity to promote and 'articulate an already-achieved gay subjectivity' that restricts and rigidifies the boundaries of the theater community itself (Joseph 2002, 109). This motivation is aptly articulated by one of Joseph's interview subjects, who viewed the theater as a valuable place for him and his partner to formulate a community of people 'like us'. In other words, his donations gave him access to people who were similarly culturally engaged:

> We had dinner with two women couples last Saturday night. One of the women is a member of the San Francisco Conservatory of Music. She loves to sing, she loves to go to the movies. We love to go to the movies. She loves to eat, we love to eat. And I guess we're sort of middle-of-the-road people. Neither one of us is flamboyantly nellie or outrageously butch. The women friends that we have would be acceptable in any company. (qtd. in Joseph 2002, 108–9)

The idea of 'acceptability' articulated here is indicative of a kind of resistance to forms of queer subjectivity that stray too far from the mainstream. The subject appears to value the fact that he and his friends live assimilative and 'middle-of-the-road' lives that give them access to the esteemed company of a member of the San Francisco Conservatory of Music, betraying an elitism that clearly grates against Prandini's purportedly 'multicultural' aims. Joseph's ethnographic research is therefore helpful in revealing how identitarian theater communities are tacitly shaped by the power of money and prevailing hegemony. Although Theatre Rhinoceros has always been a non-profit organization, the money it needs to survive is inextricably tied to donors' individual – and in this case conservative – interests.

Despite being among the most vociferously queer and counterhegemonic playwrights in the popular HIV/AIDS genre, second-generation playwrights' community orientation and lack of a universalistic and dialectical critique of hegemony's expropriative tendencies meant they often failed to address the scale of the crisis. On the one hand, their unapologetically queer dramaturgies threw a light on the suffering of HIV-positive individuals neglected by the US government and a wider constellation of right-wing culture warriors. However, as Joseph's research demonstrates, even queer theatrical institutions are vulnerable to commercial imperatives that end up reproducing normative power structures and, by extension, overlooking the need for a more universalistic politics.

Reza Abdoh: HIV/AIDS theater's peripheral vanguard

While many second-generational playwrights adopted a communitarian politics, there was at least one significant exception operating within the US HIV/AIDS genre in the 1990s. Iranian-American playwright Reza Abdoh – who died of AIDS-related causes aged 32 – produced avant-garde plays variously described as Artaudian, 'Dantesque', and 'remorseless' (Marowitz 1999, 100), and some 'of the angriest theater pieces ever hurled at a New York audience' (Holden 1999, 102). While Miller and Rudnick attempted to whip up solidaristic fervor in the auditorium, Abdoh's plays were deeply alienating in their sensorially assaultive dramaturgies, many of which addressed the AIDS crisis through visceral onstage violence, sexually explicit content, and risqué themes. At the same time, Abdoh's works retained the concoction of 'satire, farce, romance, slapstick, and burlesque' constitutive of the second-generational project; a project that thrived on experimentalism and anti-neoliberal and queer politics (Jones 1994, xi).

Perhaps the most obvious nodes of comparison between Abdoh's work and that of playwrights such as Miller relate to their vengeful and cathartic attack on US establishment representatives. Just as Jesse Helms became the subject of much of Miller's opprobrium, Abdoh featured targets for scorn throughout his oeuvre, including both explicit and thinly veiled depictions of high-profile figures. In *The*

Law of Remains (1991), for example, which tackles the government's dismissal of the AIDS crisis and the moral vapidity of contemporary media and celebrity culture, Ronald Reagan appears in the form of an inert and 'fuckable doll' (Abdoh 1996, 92). The diegesis is both phantasmagorical and absurd, representing a version of heaven occupied by Andy Warhol and Jeffrey Dahmer, the latter of whom appears to fall in a strange kind of love with the Reagan doll. To finish off the violent debasement of this much-maligned president, Abdoh's Dahmer figure describes how Reagan's post-colostomy surgery and simulated anus 'generates spontaneous orgasm in me' (Abdoh 1996, 92). Thus, the stigma and shame inflicted on America's HIV-positive constituencies by hegemonic forces is reversed back onto the US establishment – a sybaritic revenge that explicitly identifies the architects of suffering against which we must direct our ire.

However, the hopeful tenor found in Miller and Rudnick's work is markedly lacking in Abdoh's plays. Rather than rallying around an imagined 'queer community', his work delves deeper into the mucky machinations of capitalism to reveal neoliberalism's destructive impacts for racialized, gendered, poor, and sexual minority constituencies. In some ways, the experimentally protean and disjointed nature of his dramaturgy represents a fundamental tool in this exposition. Take Abdoh's production of *Bogeyman* (1991) by way of example. Staged at the Los Angeles Theater Center, the play's loose narrative follows the physical deterioration of a young man diagnosed with AIDS. Much of the play's power hinges on its set design, which includes a multi-storied cross section of an LA apartment building featuring many rooms. The play's very short scenes jump between these rooms while various screens adorn the set, encompassing a dramaturgical device that Guy Zimmerman terms 'bricolage'. Bricolage 'underscore[s] the post-punk heterogeneity and discontinuity of Abdoh's fast-paced collage aesthetic, which Marvin Carlson described as a "constant mixture of text, music, movement, video, film, and visual spectacle [...] moving so rapidly as to defy analysis, even comprehension"' (Zimmerman 2017, 62).

Such an aggressively erratic and sensorial dramaturgy forced audience members to confront the pain senselessly inflicted on those on the margins of society: the queer; HIV-positive people; sex workers; the poor. As Gautam Dasgupta notes, Abdoh's frenetic theater generated its own kind of wordless language that allowed minoritarian voices, 'unheard of within the dominant social framework', to 'seek out new models of being in the world or in a culture from which they are alienated' (Dasgupta 1994, 21). Paying little heed to the audience as consumers, Abdoh conceptualized his audience as the unwitting subjects of a neoliberal culture that blinds them to the suffering of society's economic and social underclass. His dramaturgy, then, acted as an excruciatingly visceral antidote or purgative wakeup call. As David Román noted in his review of *Bogeyman*'s production in Los Angeles, 'the sold-out run did not translate to full enthusiasm as countless subscribers walked out within the first ten minutes and missed, unfortunately, the castration-by-chainsaw scene' (Román 1992, 396). Clearly, then, Abdoh did not perceive spectators as consumers to satisfy in the way often demanded of commercial theater, but as potential antagonists to undermine in America's ongoing culture wars.

In contradistinction to the vast majority of second-generation HIV/AIDS plays, Abdoh's destabilization of spectatorial expectations allowed him to deflect conciliatory calls for communitarian pushback *within* contemporary neoliberalism's quasi-democratic order. Rather, in a way that contravenes Gramscian 'war of position' tactics, he launched wholesale attacks on the very foundations on which neoliberal subjectivity and everyday life are structured. Zimmerman's scholarship adroitly clarifies this dynamic, examining how 'Abdoh's bricolage articulates a mode of resistance to a core dynamic of neoliberalism in which the spatial conquest of industrial capitalism is transformed into a temporal form of capture' (Zimmerman 2017, 62–3). Animated by neoliberalism's overbearing productivity demands, the non-capitalist classes must devote almost every minute of their lives to marketing themselves as competitive individuals in the marketplace, crafting their lives in a strictly linear way toward either self-fulfillment or failure. If, as the old proverb goes, time is money, representing a resource that can be put toward the pursuit of profit, then scrambling time in front of audience members forces them to question the common-sense logic of rapacious neoliberal capitalism. In opposition to the unitary temporality underlying neoliberalism, Abdoh's fractured scenes represent metaphorical counterforces to the misery of the free market.

Within the context of the HIV/AIDS crisis, Abdoh's spatiotemporal experiments helped illuminate the pharmaceutical industry's culpability in prolonging pain and suffering. Toward the beginning of *Bogeyman*, a grotesque patriarch stands in front of the main apartment block, spouting offensive racial epithets and claiming to be the 'chairman of a pharmaceutical conglomerate' (Soch 2016, 00:20:00). Played by actor Tom Fitzpatrick, the patriarch is made up to appear sweaty and absurdly florid. He pats an artificially stuffed belly that protrudes so far that it cannot be mistaken for anything other than caricature, representing the greedy, nefarious nature of so-called Big

Pharma and the neoliberal American healthcare system. The play's hysterical mother character (played by Juliana Francis), meanwhile, regularly repeats 'prescribe something so I can fall asleep' (Soch 2016, 00:23:30–40), demonstrating her unwavering reliance on a system that capitalizes on addiction and suffering, as well as a critique of the nuclear familial structures vaunted by first-generation HIV/AIDS plays. The scene reaches its apogee when a writhing, lonely, and neglected AIDS patient appears onstage (played by Cliff Diller, who had advanced-stage AIDS during the performance), providing a visceral representation of the US medical establishment's inaction during the height of the crisis and, more tacitly, the wider gamut of oppressive structures perpetuated by neoliberalism.

While most of the play's scenes are very brief, the pharmaceutical chairman is permitted several minutes to rant and rave in this scene. He is also liberated from the enclosed rooms of the onstage apartment, walking freely across the entirety of the front section of the stage in a way surely symbolic of his power within the play's world of pain and corruption. He utterly monopolizes the space while reeling off a semi-comprehensible monologue that includes phrases such as 'the end is near', 'I'm gonna blow all you cocksuckers up', and 'you are all gonna die' (Soch 2016, 00:25:35–00:26:26), words reminiscent of the evangelical screeds of the American Christian Right during the 1980s and 1990s. The rant also includes mention of a so-called 'National Health Act Amendment', which promises to sterilize, maim, and abuse those of certain races or sexual orientations, or with certain diseases, as well as kill off those without health insurance, a clear allusion to the ways in which the US's privatized healthcare system renders poorer, marginalized people more vulnerable to sickness and death (Soch 2016, 00:29:32).

The outrageously violent and fascistic form of capitalism described here, combined with the temporary break from the play's customary bricolage, demonstrates the nefarious, all-consuming nature of contemporary neoliberal ideology in America, as well as its relationship with certain strata of the country's Christian Right. The fictional Health Act described by the pharmaceutical boss, for example, hints toward the relentless privatization of the healthcare sector and the consequent pricing battles that took place between pharmaceutical firms and those suffering from AIDS. Drugs company Burroughs Wellcome, for example, attracted scandal in the late 1980s after pricing the cutting-edge therapy azidothymidine (AZT) at a level that made it one of the most expensive drugs ever sold (Chase 1989). To emphasize the corrupt nature of a healthcare system that brazenly favors the lives and wellbeing of the rich, *Bogeyman*'s pharmaceutical chairman stands outside of the apartment block while delivering his speech. He has the privilege of looking at the world (or, at least, the diegesis of the play) in its entirety, addressing other characters who can see him but not each other. This affords him a sort of power with which he can manipulate and control the subjugated characters of the play, dictating which spaces they are allowed to occupy and controlling the information to which they are exposed. The character of the pharmaceutical chairman, then, is a physically rendered metaphor for the power of a market-driven society to oppress its poorer or less 'desirable' members. For people with AIDS, whose lives were already devalued by dint of stigma and widespread homophobia, the option to receive treatment lay solely with the moneyed.

Since Abdoh's death in 1995, the HIV/AIDS genre has failed to throw up such eye-openingly visceral and anti-capitalist work, at least in the commercial theaters of the Global North. Perhaps critic, director, and playwright Charles Marowitz put it best, writing in a review of *Bogeyman*, 'No matter how much we distract ourselves from the fact, the AIDS epidemic is an inescapable reality, and the superstitious desire to relegate it to one segment of the population cannot prevent us from stumbling over the corpses or getting the stench of deadly tumescence in our nostrils' (Marowitz 1999, 100). As we will briefly touch on in the following chapter, Abdoh was one of a very small number of playwrights of color who addressed the racial politics of the epidemic in America and attempted to reveal the full extent of the crisis. Combining humor, shock tactics, and a materialist dramaturgy, Abdoh's work occupied its own unique space within a second generation of playwrights myopically fighting for a subsection of gay, middle-class America. For this reason, his work warrants renewed scholarly attention.

CHAPTER THREE

Race and Absence in HIV/AIDS Theater

Ever since the HIV/AIDS crisis was brought to public attention in the early 1980s, related cultural production in the Global North has overwhelmingly focused on the lives of young, white, gay men. Given the ubiquity of such whitewashed (or, as discussed in Chapter 1, 'nostalgic') narratives, non-experts in the history and politics of HIV/AIDS would be forgiven for assuming the crisis is 1) virtually over, 2) largely confined to white, queer constituencies, and 3) increasingly untethered from political struggle in contemporary society. None of these notions could be further from the truth, as the pandemic continues to disproportionately affect poor and marginalized peoples throughout the world. As I write this, the latest statistics from UNAIDS state that there are over 37 million people living with HIV worldwide, over a quarter of whom are not accessing antiretroviral treatment (HIV.gov 2022). In the US, the highest infection rate pertained to the Black population (42.1%), followed by the Latinx population (21.7%), demonstrating the extent to which HIV/AIDS disproportionately affects racialized communities (HIV.gov 2021). Perhaps predictably given the country's hyper-marketized healthcare system, the US represents one of the more extreme exemplars of inequity surrounding HIV/AIDS care in the Global North. As such, this chapter will zone in on US histories and texts to exemplify neoliberalism's role in perpetuating HIV/AIDS crises among racialized groups while erasing their members' experiences from mainstream cultural narratives.

Fortunately, the political valences surrounding infection rates are garnering ever more attention in HIV/AIDS humanities scholarship, and the field is generating new frameworks for understanding how cultural narratives surrounding the pandemic are fomented. As noted in Chapter 1, Jih-Fei Cheng et al.'s *AIDS and the Distribution of Crises* (2020) represents one of the most comprehensive multiple-authored volumes to disrupt orthodox understanding of HIV/AIDS, ultimately positing that 'AIDS is not a crisis. It is a global distribution of networked crises', the most neglected of which are brimming with uncharted perspectives and subjects (Cheng et al. 2020, 17). Robb Hernandez's *Archiving an Epidemic: Art, AIDS, and the Queer Chicanx Avant-Garde* (2019), meanwhile, attempts to reconstruct histories of HIV/AIDS in Chicanx communities through examination of archived artworks and the deployment of so-called 'queer detrital analysis', working to fill epistemic gaps generated by the erasure of Chicanx cultural products. Dan Royles' *To Make the Wounded Whole: The African American Struggle Against HIV/AIDS* (2020) is also instructive, working to reveal underexamined histories of Black HIV/AIDS activism in the US and countering narratives that posit white, queer populations as primary drivers of change. While this valuable scholarship is working to change hegemonic narratives, it remains the case that racial disparities surrounding the pandemic are systematically underreported and therefore underappreciated in the public consciousness. As such, given this volume's politico-economic orientation, I will briefly summarize the ways in which neoliberal hegemonic forces have worked to obfuscate and compound the spread of HIV/AIDS in racialized communities in the Global North since the pandemic began. Then, I will explain how such a dynamic links to the broader neoliberalization of theater, the whitewashing of the HIV/AIDS genre, and the recent emergence of plays that examine HIV/AIDS in Black communities while adhering to distinctly neoliberal public health paradigms.

Capitalism, race, and HIV/AIDS in America

One of the first major scholarly works to explore the political and social impacts of HIV/AIDS on America's Black populations was Cathy Cohen's *The Boundaries of Blackness: AIDS and the Breakdown of Black Politics* (1999). Offering a comprehensive overview of the ways in which the pandemic compounded existing political tensions among different marginalized groups, Cohen's work demonstrated how issues surrounding class and sexuality operated alongside racism to conceal the extent to which HIV/AIDS affected Black populations during the 1980s and 1990s. The book remains instructive today, particularly for those hoping to make sense of the overwhelming whiteness of cultural production surrounding HIV/AIDS in the US. While this phenomenon was undoubtedly overdetermined, Cohen partly explains such stark misrepresentation through sophisticated mechanisms of marginalization unique to capitalist modes of production – sometimes referred to as 'racial capitalism'. Commonly attributed to Cedric Robinson's *Black Marxism* (1983), the term 'racial capitalism' has recently gained ground as a means to overcome debates about the role of class and/or identity in the formation of oppressive structures by positing racism as a requisite component of capitalist production. While all forms of capitalism necessarily involve racialization, the term is useful in drawing attention to the expropriative function of a system that denies the oppressive foundations of its existence.

Before discussing the merits of Cohen's work, it might be helpful to provide readers with an overview of how racial capitalism and marginalization operate under the current socio-economic order. While neoliberal ideologues tend to sell the so-called 'free' market as a racial leveler offering social mobility for those willing to work hard, its measurable and all-too-blatant effects tell a very different story. Michael C. Dawson and Megan Ming Francis, along with an increasing number of political theorists, deploy the term 'racial capitalism' to describe the continued exploitation and expropriation of Black populations following the dismantling of Jim Crow restrictions. Both point to phenomena such as the war on drugs, the proliferation of cheap prison labor, high incarceration rates, and the criminalization of private debt as capitalism's ostensibly 'color-blind' methods for maintaining and reproducing white supremacy in the US. Lacking the capital necessary to join the ranks of the white middle classes, already immiserated Black populations have been continually expropriated by such systems for decades. At the same time, hegemonic powers have worked to naturalize disproportionately high rates of poverty and incarceration among racialized communities in a bid to quell dissent and secure consent for the actions of the neoliberal state. More specifically, a small number of Black elites have been elevated into positions of power under late capitalism, lending credibility to its fictions of social mobility at the same time as vast swathes of the Black lower classes have been cast as 'undeserving' of state assistance or financial redress. Indeed, 'particularly susceptible to neoliberal arguments were black leaders, intellectuals, and organizations that either were predisposed or came to believe that cultural pathologies of the underclass were substantially responsible for persisting black inequalities' (Dawson and Francis 2015, 44).

As the 2020s push on and neoliberalism rapidly evolves in a bid to weather heightening crises and contradictions, such racial dynamics grow ever more intense. As Arun Kundnani explains in his critique of Friedrich Hayek's theory of cultural evolution, neoliberalism is constituted in such a way that it requires racism for its very subsistence. Reflecting on the intensification of populist rhetoric surrounding border regimes in recent years, Kundnani rejects the idea that such racialized dogma is employed simply to displace hostility toward neoliberalism's inequities onto convenient scapegoats. Citing work by the likes of Wendy Brown and David Harvey, he asserts that some of today's most prolific political economists interpret racism as a vestigial element of a previous, brutal era that tends to emerge as a cultural backlash against neoliberal cosmopolitanism. For Kundnani, however, populist politics 'can only be made sense of by understanding the "material and social base" of actual racial divisions of labour and the racist practices of neoliberal states, which provide a legitimacy and spontaneous "folk" plausibility to right-wing racist rhetoric' (Kundnani 2021, 66). The global policing of migrants, for example, is a crucial tool for neoliberal states to deal with 'surplus populations' and maintain divisions of labor that ensure that Global South populations remain readily exploitable and far away from the wealth accrued by Global North states. So, recent electoral successes by overtly racist politicians do not represent a significant shift away from the core functions of neoliberalism – they simply lay bare the racial ordering upon which neoliberalism has always relied. It is against such a socio-economic environment and trajectory, that we must analyze the racial politics of HIV/AIDS in the US and, indeed, the rest of the Global North. While it might feel easy or logical to dismiss the absence of racial minorities onstage as the fault of elitist theaters pushing out artists of color – or, indeed, homophobia within certain marginalized groups – the racism churning under the surface of neoliberalism has necessarily shaped political and artistic responses to the crisis in ways that warrant exploration, careful articulation, and pushback.

With this in mind, let us return to Cohen's exploration of Black responses to HIV/AIDS. During Reagan's administration, she notes, the president legitimized his opposition to race-specific welfare policies and healthcare provisions by appointing Black conservatives to positions of power, thus obscuring the role of neoliberalism in compounding socio-economic inequalities along racial lines. At the same time, Black community leaders gravitated toward advocating for the 'innocent victims' of the crisis (such as children), wary as they were of the ways in which sexual stereotypes were used to justify the continued impoverishment of racialized groups – seen, for example, in Reagan's flagrant deployment of the sexualized 'welfare queen' trope. Therefore, claims Cohen, the limited institutional responses that emerged out of Black communities were primarily centered on education and prevention services. While this work was spearheaded primarily by Black gay men and lesbians motivated by the urgency of the crisis, it lacked 'the more aggressive political tactics of civil disobedience used by predominantly white groups such as ACT UP', focusing on compromise and education rather than confronting oppressive structures (Cohen 1999, 340–1). Unlike many of ACT UP's white members, Black activists faced a multiplicity of obstacles that hindered progress and stemmed from prejudices extending far beyond homophobia. A corollary of the racialized dispossession outlined above was the invisibilizing of marginalized peoples with AIDS to institutions such as the Centers for Disease Control and Prevention (CDC). Lacking adequate access to healthcare, many of their deaths were not recorded as AIDS-related, meaning the spread of the pandemic among these populations went untracked. As Cohen explains, such underreporting meant that 'Black communities did not identify with those considered to be at risk, so did not think of themselves as susceptible to infection' (Cohen 1999, 139).

Compounding this lack of material care and attention was a spirit of social conservativism that ran through pockets of Black America. On top of the homophobia that came out of Black church-going communities, the crisis enflamed and ignited intra-racial prejudices toward marginalized groups such as drug users and the poor. Much of Cohen's book analyzes the role popular media sources such as newspapers and magazines played in fomenting common-sense ideas about HIV/AIDS within racialized communities. Indeed, her project reflects a kind of Gramscian mindedness in this respect, convinced as she was that cultural production represents a tool in the constant tussle over hegemonic dominance between different groups in society and, therefore, is inextricably tied to questions of political economy. Of course, Gramsci cannot straightforwardly be described as a scholar of racism or imperialism, focused as he was on intra-European politics and culture. However, as Stuart Hall noted in the 1990s, Gramsci's characterization of hegemony as a complex system of alliances that cannot be explained by class division alone represents a fertile theoretical lens through which to analyze antagonisms and divisions within subaltern groups. By analyzing how contemporary ideological terrains are constructed by interactions and expedient deals made between seemingly hostile forces and institutions – such as ethnically specific media outlets, schools, churches, cultural organizations, and more – we might start to understand how, for example, the demonization of the Black 'underclass' and 'welfare queens' incentivized a kind of respectability politics in the Black press that allowed the epidemic to go underreported and misunderstood. In short, a Gramscian framework focused on analyzing and interpreting the wider implications of cultural production 'helps us to understand one of the most common, least explained features of "racism"; the "subjection" of the victims of racism to the mystifications of the very racist ideologies which imprison and define them' (Hall 1996, 440).

The best example of this obfuscatory function is the volume of media coverage centered on Earvin 'Magic' Johnson, a world-famous basketball player who announced his seropositive status in 1991. The news forced media outlets who had been silent on the issue of HIV/AIDS in Black communities to start acknowledging the need for improved healthcare and research. However, Johnson's revelation was quickly followed by reassurances of his heterosexuality and moralistic statements about the need for young people to remain abstinent – a tacit form of homophobia that 'exacerbated the dominant media's dodging of what some might consider the "seamier" side of AIDS in black communities' (Cohen 1999, 149). Of all the stories covering AIDS and Black communities published in *The New York Times* between 1981 and 1993, 49% were about Magic Johnson and a further 13% were about Arthur Ashe, another Black sportsman who contracted HIV from a blood transfusion (Cohen 1999, 161). Portrayed as straight, successful, and family-oriented, these celebrities were viewed as deserving recipients of public sympathy. Rather than galvanizing discussions surrounding the need to fund research and healthcare for poor and queer Black Americans with HIV, these cases compounded existing stigmas within the Black community and wider America. This pattern is, of course, consistent with neoliberalism's atomistic imperative for self-sufficiency and nuclear familial ties, as well as the hegemonic tactic that elevates a small number of Black individuals to the detriment of immiserated populations. Even those nominally on the side of the most marginalized in society – such as the 'paucity of leftist journals and magazines' aimed at the Black community – failed to criticize some of the demonizing narratives espoused by Black conservative institutions and elected officials (Cohen 1999, 239). Wary of alienating themselves from the Black political class, leftists engaged in 'a strategy of constructive engagement [...] to deal with the "mainstream" of the black community' (Cohen 1999, 243). As such, the extent of pain and suffering in America's racialized communities remained – and, to a large extent, still remains – invisible.

Before we return to the question of theater, it is worth acknowledging that subcultural and countercultural projects of resistance have existed throughout Black America since the early years of the epidemic – despite an overwhelmingly hostile sociopolitical environment. While Cohen gestures toward such groups in *The Boundaries of Blackness*, Dan Royles' more recent work offers a wider conspectus of activism, artwork, and community projects surrounding Black Americans affected by the epidemic. Emphasizing the various ways in which Black AIDS activists faced greater challenges relative to their white counterparts, Royles argues that such adversity bestowed upon them a greater understanding of the structural inequities undergirding the crisis. ACT UP Philadelphia, for example, which contained a much higher proportion of Black members than other chapters around the country, pushed for global access to effective therapies in a bid to address AIDS as 'a problem of inequality' inextricably bound to histories of plunder, 'from the European empires that grew rich off the labor of enslaved Africans to the multinational corporations that dominate global markets' (Royles 2020, 7). While Cohen's book focuses on the ways in which dominant hegemonic forces fractured Black politics, Royles' work explores how grassroots subcultural responses to the crisis ignited new coalitions and systems of political thought within small pockets of America. Throughout the rest of this chapter, I will ensure that such hopeful or reparative phenomena remain within our field of vision, while critiquing the relatively barren landscape of mainstream HIV/AIDS theater produced by dramaturgs of color. In so doing, I hope to demonstrate both the power of capitalistic forces in keeping a vast nexus of marginalized voices from entering public consciousness and the determination of these activists and creatives to continue their work despite such adversity.

Race and American HIV/AIDS theater in the 'crisis years'

As explored in the previous chapter, Reza Abdoh was arguably one of the most widely recognized playwrights of color on the American theater scene to address the intersecting politics of race and HIV/AIDS. While the majority of widely publicized HIV/AIDS plays focused on the lives of relatively moneyed gay men, works such as Abdoh's *The Law of Remains* (1992) punctured the homogeneity of the off-Broadway landscape and its equivalents outside of New York. The play comprises a partial retelling of the infamous Jeffrey Dahmer murders, comparing governmental and media indifference and lack of compassion toward Dahmer's queer victims of color to the similarly pitiful and prejudicial responses to the AIDS crisis. Like Cohen, Abdoh was keen to highlight how institutions within the news media generate and affirm consent for the dehumanization of society's racialized constituencies. Ever the provocateur, he was free to use the stage as a medium through which to galvanize political awareness of racial capitalism's effects through horror-inflected esthetics.

Throughout *The Law of Remains*, Dahmer's character (named Jeffrey Snarling) is accompanied by Warhola, a caricatured Andy Warhol intent on creating a sensationalist documentary about Snarling's crimes to 'make a heap of money' (Abdoh 1996, 82). The voyeuristic presence of Warhola encourages the sprawling discussion of Dahmer's crimes to become increasingly lewd, scandalmongering, and laden with slurs – an execrable bid to generate profit-worthy spectacle. At one point, a character reels off the names, ages, and racial identities of Dahmer's real-life victims, while Snarling chimes in with such remorseless comments as 'Lean, sick junkies under my cleaver. I'll relieve them. Soft sadness of death' and 'The cow god, the horse god, the bank god, the cop god claim their yearly crop. This is America' (Abdoh 1996, 83) – a reference, surely, to law enforcement's complicity as a node in the system of racial capitalism. In describing the deaths of marginalized citizens as a 'yearly crop' expunged from society by functionaries of the state, Snarling lays bare the ways in which the banalization of violence upholds contemporary systems of expropriation and capitalist profiteering by hegemonic means.

As Joseph Cermatori explains, in such moments 'the AIDS crisis comes into view as a political, spiritual, and moral crisis in which the lives of outsiders are devalued and mocked' (Cermatori 2020, 132). Far from representing the *symptoms* or *unplanned consequences* of the capitalist mode of production, the mutilated bodies of Dahmer's victims are – as theorists of racial capitalism would attest – intentionally woven into its very fabric. The murder of young queer boys of color

> provides a continual down payment so that Warhol's art market, like all other newly unfettered markets, can operate. The homophobic society of 1980s America could only continue conducting business as usual by rendering invisible the human cost of the AIDS epidemic, all while it also produced an ongoing media spectacle via television airwaves [...] *The Law of Remains* exposes the banality by which capitalism and violence toward socially precarious "unmentionables" – members of

> minority groups, migrants, the diseased, disabled, and poor – go hand in hand. (Cermatori 2020, 132)

In viscerally exposing this mutually reinforcing relationship, Abdoh stood out from many of the HIV/AIDS playwrights who gained similar levels of exposure. While nostalgic plays were frequently praised for their ability to spark audiences' empathic capacities, Abdoh's work forced critics and spectators to confront the structural and hegemonic factors that prolonged the HIV/AIDS crisis. A review acknowledging the play's purpose as a 'metaphor for governmental indifference to the AIDS crisis' (Holden 1999, 102), for example, found an unlikely platform in *The New York Times*, a newspaper frequently condemned by AIDS activists for its refusal to publish sufficient content about the epidemic (art collective Gran Fury even produced a satirical paper entitled *The New York Crimes* to express their disgust with the organization's response). Clearly, therefore, the play managed to cut through established institutional boundaries and subvert hegemonic narratives in a way that few of Abdoh's contemporaries could have hoped to achieve.

While much of Abdoh's work has garnered scholarly praise for its excoriating critique of racism in America, however, I would be remiss not to mention some of the more controversial or misguided dramaturgical techniques Abdoh employed to shine a light on racial inequities. The best example of such notorious theater-making is *Tight Right White* (1993). Loosely based on *Mandingo* (1975), a blaxploitation film about the treatment of enslaved people in the antebellum South, it brazenly plays with a cornucopia of garish stereotypes and assaults its audience with Abdoh's signature orgiastic style. White actors in blackface deal and shoot drugs, Black actors in white makeup chant Nazi slogans and taunt and dehumanize white actors, Klan members dance around waving Confederate flags, and a Jewish TV producer named Moishe Pipik attempts to profit from the mayhem while exhibiting a host of antisemitic stereotypes, including a prosthetic hooked nose and a fixation on a magical money tree. The show's reviewers were unanimous in their conviction that the show was risky and jarring, and purposely alienated the theatergoing public. Writing in the *Village Voice*, renowned critic Michael Feingold dubbed *Tight Right White* a 'psychological enema, shoved up the id of liberal theatergoers to expel the unhealthy imprints a racist society has deposited there', while speculating that 'African, Asian, Jewish, and gay Americans would fail to see anything in his work but a hideous outpouring of filth' (Feingold 1999, 104).

It certainly seems unlikely that such offensive racial imagery would make it onto today's stage. As Tobi Haslett notes in a recent reappraisal of the play,

> a contemporary critic can only sigh, and say – so much of *Tight Right White* is impossible to justify. Its gestures violate the standards of our day, and of Abdoh's. Whether intended as metaphor or as gimmick or as theory of pop, there's no satirical inflection or grandiloquent irony that can contain or nullify the force of blackface. (Haslett n.d.)

However, Haslett also remarks that most people can never hope to understand the play's affective force, having not been in the auditorium. He continues,

> There are scripts and bleary videos of *Tight Right White*, yes, but they muffle the blast of the thing they seek to save. The hunger and hurt of this dead man's play lie at an elaborate remove, now, from who and what I am – my bouquet of identities and tastes – but whatever that is owes something to what he did. He can madden and offend me, transfix and perplex me. But he eludes me. (Haslett n.d.)

Such ambivalence reflects, perhaps, the way in which many critics' feelings of visceral disgust competed with the suspicion that Abdoh's assaultive techniques offer something of a political force for good. In a bid to make sense of *Tight Right White*'s counterhegemonic potential, for example, Ehren Fordyce applies Jose Esteban Muñoz's notion of 'disidentification' to an optimistic analysis of the play's politics. Muñoz describes disidentification as a technique that scrambles and reconstructs encoded messages within cultural products in a way that 'exposes the encoded message's universalizing and exclusionary machination and recircuits its workings to account for, include, and empower minority identities and identifications' (Muñoz 1999, 31). Thus, Abdoh's cross-racial and cross-gender casting 'plays against the lack of slippage, or "tightness", in such identifications [of whiteness as mastery and the dark other as queer and submissive], creating at least some possibility for moving away from, or at least not being reduced to, these symptoms of the American imaginary' (Fordyce 2004, 224). In other words, the offensive and assaultive imagery serves a kind of expurgatory purpose, moving beyond the messy strictures of identity to open up new pathways to solidarity.

Clearly, unraveling the affective and galvanizing dimensions of *Tight Right White* is an endlessly complex task that lies outside the scope of my analysis. While we might read any of Abdoh's plays as reacting to the hegemonic narratives and structural inequities that compounded the oppression of HIV-positive people in the 1980s and 1990s, *Tight Right White* does not directly address the HIV/AIDS crisis in the same way as *Bogeyman* or *The Law of Remains*. As such, I will not explore *Tight Right White* in further detail. I have offered a brief overview of this most audacious and perhaps injudicious of works not to loosen the definitional strictures of the HIV/ADS play, but to emphasize the fragile ground upon which Abdoh trod as an HIV-positive playwright staging risky political work in mainstream auditoria. In one sense, challenging and undermining the racist stereotypes that undergird hegemonic narratives necessitates the creation of something bold, pioneering, and discomfiting. However, Abdoh's decision to embrace and intensify the sexualized stereotypes that threatened activists of color seeking dignity, healthcare, and attention might easily be read as counterintuitive. I question the wisdom of making flesh the phantasmic prejudices of the most hardened edges of America's evangelical right and allowing them to run riot, especially with the culture wars raging. As Joshua Chambers-Letson notes, 'Though [Abdoh's] intention clearly seems to the contrary, his work often offers less a cogent critique of antiblack racism than a frantic, exhausted, hopeless, and fleshy rearticulation of it', citing a review by eminent critic Charles Marowitz as a case in point (Chambers-Letson 2018). For Marowitz, Abdoh's oeuvre served to depict 'a drug-addled, plague-ridden, crime-infested society that nightly reports the murders and atrocities of a civilization going down the tubes' (Marowitz 1999, 99). Employing the stigmatizing and dehumanizing language of the dominant hegemonic order ('drug-addled', 'plague-ridden', 'crime-infested'), Marowitz views the play as affirming right-wing fears surrounding the supposed 'invasion' of Black and brown subjects and the degradation of a Western imperialist conception of 'civilization'.

It is also worth noting that, as an Iranian-American primarily working between New York and Los Angeles, Abdoh operated within a political and social sphere substantially different from those invisibilized and oppressed constituencies also affected by HIV/AIDS – namely, Black Americans. While acutely aware of the racial capitalist system on which America rested, Abdoh was not subject to the deep intra-community divisions Cohen's work emphasizes. Taking Philadelphia as an example, Royles explains that the city's history of racism and segregation meant that sexual identities and subcultures within its respective white and Black communities were very different. While downtown Philadelphia contained a largely white, gay enclave,

'Black gay men and women tended to live in neighborhoods defined by race rather than sexuality' (Royles 2020, 46). As such, communal identities and spatial politics shaped the tactics of Black artists and grassroots movements, many of which were forced to confront both homophobic attitudes within communities of color and racist attitudes within white gay and minority AIDS agencies (Royles 2020, 33). The Gay Men of Color Consortium (GMOCC), for example, believed in providing safe sex education that boosted the self-esteem of gay and bisexual Black men as a starting point for reducing infection rates (Royles 2020, 59). Meanwhile, sexual health advocates staged educative plays such as *Choices* – a didactic piece about teenage sexuality and the AIDS crisis by the group Blacks Educating Blacks About Sexual Health Issues (BEBASHI) (Royles 2020, 35). Rather than confront the overwhelming and complex modes of domination that rendered racialized populations more vulnerable to HIV, these organizations and activists focused on developing support networks and education programs within their communities. While it is unclear how such organizations and activists would have received a play such as Abdoh's *Tight Right White* or *The Law of Remains*, the chasm between their consciousness-raising and mitigative tactics is clear.

Of course, there are limitations to adopting what we might refer to as 'standpoint epistemology' here – that is, the notion that marginalized constituencies have unique access to knowledge about their social position and the nature of their oppression and, therefore, are better placed to produce salient critiques or solutions. As philosopher Olúfẹ́mi O. Táíwò has explained, such a political orientation might be counterintuitive in certain contexts, given the ways in which capitalism works to locate 'attentional injustice in the selection of spokespeople and book lists taken to represent the marginalized, rather than focusing on the action of the corporations and algorithms that much more powerfully distribute attention' (Táíwò 2022, 72). The theater might represent a particularly good example of an institution that strategically platforms the voices of the more moneyed or advantageously networked echelons of a given minoritarian constituency, erroneously presenting these figures as reliable representatives of a whole group while capitalizing on the considerable reputational advantages that come with diversifying once-homogeneous sites of social influence. Elite capture, as Táíwò names this phenomenon, 'directs what little attentional power we can control at symbolic sites of power rather than at the root political issues that explain why everything is so fucked up' (Táíwò 2022, 72).

Certainly, it can be helpful to remind ourselves of the power of elite capture when analyzing the politics of contemporary theater in commercial and state-subsidized institutions, particularly given the intensification of profit-making imperatives generated by neoliberal hegemony. However, given the extent to which HIV/AIDS playwrights were often closely involved with, or at least exposed to, socially situated grassroots movements during the last decades of the twentieth century, standpoint epistemology might offer an elucidatory framework through which to identify *some* of the potential oversights or epistemic lacunae in works such as Abdoh's. I turn now, therefore, to one of the few counterhegemonic Black theater groups to have tackled the politics of HIV/AIDS on the mainstream stage, in contradistinction to the community and outreach-oriented works already mentioned. Active in the early 1990s when HIV/AIDS theater took on its more counterhegemonic edge, the Pomo Afro Homos (or Postmodern African American Homosexuals) were a collective who performed in major theaters in San Francisco, New York, and London, in universities, and even on *Oprah*. Initially, the troupe consisted of Djola Bernard Branner, Brian Freeman, and Eric Gupton, although they were later joined by Marvin K. White. Having gained recognition relatively quickly, the Pomos used their platform to raise audiences' consciousness of both racism in the gay community and homophobia in the Black community, often with a keen eye on how these seemingly unrelated forces stemmed from broader political phenomena that were prolonging the HIV/AIDS crisis.

One of the group's most popular and comedically acerbic pieces was *Dark Fruit* (1994), a series of skits that satirized and critiqued powerful groups or individuals who were quietly failing to stand by Black queer people in the midst of a deadly epidemic. The first sketch in the play, titled 'Aunties in America', represents a brief parody of Kushner's *Angels in America*, teasing out moments in which Kushner falls into prejudicial or politically myopic traps. While I launched a critical defense of *Angels* against some of its best-known detractors earlier in this book, it is worth returning to the weaker elements of the play's racial politics to uncover how they might have alienated Black or minority audience members – and, therefore, to understand how the more general whiteness of HIV/AIDS theater might have produced antagonisms counter to a solidaristic politics.

By far the most widely cited issue identified with Kushner's play is the treatment of the character Belize, whose role as a nurse, faithful friend, and thankless confidante has garnered condemnation for embodying a so-called 'Magical Negro' stereotype – in other words, a Black character whose sole purpose is to fulfill the emotional and physical needs of white protagonists while giving little away about their own thoughts, feelings, or desires. When the most recent revival of *Angels* hit London's National Theatre in 2017 and New York's Broadway the following year, much of the more censorious press coverage surrounding the play focused on the perpetuation of this trope. Writing for *BuzzFeed News*, scholar Steven W. Thrasher identified *Angels'* racial politics as its most 'unforgivable' aspect, condemning the role of Belize as a 'male mammy who exists primarily to develop white characters emotionally and enlighten white audiences', employing the logic of standpoint epistemology to support this critique. As a queer person of color, Thrasher registers his discomfort with much of the play, particularly

> when Belize and Louis are on a bench and Louis is talking — and talking, and talking, ejaculating a monologue of bullshit at Belize while the black character throws shade in looks. When I saw it, the overwhelmingly white audience found this hilarious. But if you're a queer of color and have ever been spoken to in this way, you don't find Louis very funny. (Thrasher 2018)

In Chapter 1, I examined the ways in which this scene propelled what I conceptualize as the play's core internal dialectic, which asks audience members to see past vacuous axioms of solidarity to consider the tussle between the experiential knowledge of those suffering most intensely in Reagan's America and the assertions of those free to intellectualize such misery. Through this lens, it is difficult to see how such a scene could be interpreted as light relief or comedy. However, given Belize's established role as the 'Magical Negro', in which he neatly mops up the mistakes of the play's flawed white liberals, I have sympathy for the notion that Kushner's complex and ambivalent treatment of the meaning of 'progress' and identity might be undermined by the more reductive aspects of Belize's character. As the elusive and entertaining 'mammy' figure, Belize represents a repository for white liberal guilt, generating a kind of affective catharsis that cleanses the audience's white members of their potential discomfort and flips it back onto queers of color, such as Thrasher.

In a bid to highlight this affective function, the Pomos' parodic version of *Angels* replaces white protagonist Prior with Belize in one of the play's pivotal scenes, when an angel crashes through the ceiling to deliver a prophetic message. Rather than faithfully replicate Prior's epiphanic moment, Belize breaks character in a comedic moment of metatheater, as two spectators – Paul and Jacob – watch on. He asks the pair why 'Missy Kushner has me up there every night reading these white kids' asses or wiping their butts. It's all the same to me. In part two I get to wipe Roy Cohn's butt. Find an epiphany in that!' (Pomo Afro Homos 2018, 324). In overlooking what might be read as the more profound or political elements of the play, the Pomos revel in toilet humor, pointing out the fairly crude ways in which Kushner's play degrades its characters of color via the visceral perpetuation of regressive stereotypes. While the play's characters grapple with abstract and weighty questions surrounding capitalism, religion, humanity's progress, and more, Belize carries out much of the socially reproductive work which makes such intellectual activity possible. In pointing out this subjugative relation, the troupe undermine the pedestal on which 'Missy Kushner' was placed following the overwhelming success of *Angels*, which had already received a string of high-profile industry awards by the time *Dark Fruit* was premiered, including a Pulitzer Prize for Drama.

Such remonstrances are not leveled at Kushner alone, however, as Belize, Paul, and Jacob (all actors) rant about the indignities to which other Broadway playwrights have subjected their Black characters. John Guare is a target of Paul's ire, for example, as he explains:

> Belize, I know what you mean about them trying to find their epiphanies through us. You see, Missy Guare has me up there with all these Upper East Side most worrisome white folks, processing all their yap-de-yap get-a-clue-already angst. Then I have to feed 'em. Then I have to fuck 'em. (Pomo Afro Homos 2018, 324)

He is, presumably, critiquing Guare's critically lauded *Six Degrees of Separation* (1990) here, a play about a Black gay conman who schemes his way into admittance into the social milieu of New York's white elite, another example of work in which a sole Black character is planted to represent the needs and concerns of an entire racial group in a bid to enlighten a group of clueless, moneyed liberals. Given how capitalism's survival relies on new and established forms of racism, however, the actors are caught in a double bind regarding their role within theatrical institutions and as workers more generally. Confronting the possibility of opting out of capitalist modes of production, Belize exclaims, 'But what we gonna do? Quit?' and the group members '*all laugh an over-the-top laugh*' (Pomo Afro Homos 2018, 325), a cynical expression of the ways in which capitalism forces workers to abnegate their convictions in exchange for the material resources necessary for survival. So long as white theater makers hold the lion's share of capital channeled into producing mainstream shows, they imply, Black voices and perspectives will remain ancillary. Certainly, this dynamic ensured that all of the best-known HIV/AIDS plays produced during the early years of the crisis elevated the experiences of a relatively small, wealthy subsection of society. For all the staunchly anti-Republican sentiment that roils through Kushner's play, the Pomos' problematization of its racial homogeneity and capitulation to stigmatizing norms elucidates the ways in which a truly solidaristic and effective anti-capitalist theater requires a nuanced and careful approach to the depiction of race relations onstage. Whether a play with such a politics could ever find its way into mainstream theaters while such institutions remain in thrall to capitalistic imperatives is, of course, an unresolved question.

The Pomos do not reserve their ire for whiteness and racial capitalism alone, however. The final sketch of *Dark Fruit*, titled 'Chocolate City USA', represents an angrier reproach of groups and individuals beyond the cozy liberal confines of the theater. Set in the midst of the National March on Washington for Lesbian and Gay Rights, the performer reads out a series of letters condemning the media, the CDC, Black Gay Men, the Clintons, Black churches, AIDS organizations including Gay Men's Health Crisis and ACT UP, and, simply, America for failing to address the HIV/AIDS crisis in Black communities. Perhaps the strongest critique is saved for basketball superstar Magic Johnson, whose HIV diagnosis dominated news coverage about HIV/AIDS in Black populations in the US in the early 1990s. Despite Johnson's activism and HIV advocacy work, the Pomos address him as follows: 'Dear Magic, Heroes are like fast food; they always disappoint. You write a book that nobody reads. You make a video that nobody watches. You start another celebrity AIDS foundation that nobody needs. You were the cure. Magic. Right? You were. Now you're a sportscaster. What happened?' (Pomo Afro Homos 2018, 341). What the troupe hint at here are the ideological undercurrents of Johnson's advocacy work, which saw him continually reiterate his heterosexuality, promote abstinence among young people, and obscure the scale of the epidemic among Black people in the US. Johnson stood in as a hegemonic tool of the dominant classes, rigidifying repressive sexual norms and leaving insurgent activists and artists such as the Afro Pomo Homos with the insurmountable task of sticking up for the stigmatized and the dispossessed in the midst of crisis.

For the Pomos, any emancipatory project fighting for the lives of all HIV-positive people required a kind of fearlessness that many Black AIDS organizations and community groups were lacking. As they impatiently intone in 'Chocolate City USA', 'Dear Black Gay Men, I am fed up with going to demonstrations without you, then listening to you complain about the white boys that did. Isn't that closet getting kind cramped?' (Pomo Afro Homos 2018, 341). In contradistinction to the cautious approach adopted by some Black churches and AIDS organizations, many of which attempted to protect themselves from stigmatizing narratives surrounding promiscuity and drug-taking, one of the Pomos ends *Dark Fruit* by emphasizing: 'Engrave on my tombstone/ "Here sleeps a *happy* black faggot/ Who lived to love and died/ With no guilt"' (Pomo Afro Homos 2018, 343). The frustration and fortitude clearly undergirding this sentiment, combined with repeated material demands that 'We need equal access to drugs and treatment' (Pomo Afro Homos 2018, 343), reflects an understanding of capitalism and stigma as inextricably entwined.

As Imogen Tyler expounds in her extensive exploration of the political economy of stigma, the propagation of dehumanizing narratives about subsections of society cannot be satisfactorily comprehended through psychological and social scientific frameworks divorced from power relations. Zoning in on twenty-first-century Britain by way of example, Tyler explains that the dehumanization of the country's poor as 'benefit scroungers' (and other variations on this theme) reflects 'a political programme that involves the fracking of public goods by those in the service of capital, in ways that are designed to upend the customary forms of social provision cemented in the mid-twentieth century' (Tyler 2020, 170). Without monstering the group from which such goods were pilfered, the dominant powers would likely have experienced destabilizing pushback by prosocial and ethical tendencies within the wider citizenry. For neoliberalism to shore up consensus and maintain its hegemony, instilling a fear of (and a fear of becoming) an 'other' was essential for retaining power over the most marginalized groups on which relentless production and unbridled capitalist growth rely, especially as the conventions of our financialized economy allow the gulf between rich and poor to grow. In late twentieth-century America, this relation was perfectly exemplified by the culture warriors of the right and their use of stigmatizing invectives against marginalized groups, including both Black people and the queer. The Pomos were acutely aware of this relation, and their playtexts and theatrical recordings are vital reminders that – while small – there existed a vanguard of dramaturgs within the HIV/AIDS genre willing to explicitly condemn a host of (often disparate, sometimes even liberal-minded) forces curtailing the ability of racialized people to access HIV/AIDS treatments and care.

Finally, before we move onto examining twenty-first-century theater, I will briefly mention another member of this marginalized vanguard, albeit they are less well-known than the Pomos. Rhodessa Jones is an actress, teacher, and writer known for setting up the Medea Project, a performance workshop designed to help incarcerated women navigate the social and personal challenges associated with HIV diagnosis. In 1997, Jones performed a short solo piece, *Deep in the Night*, at the African American Performance Art Festival in New York. Conceived as a means to open up public dialogue about HIV/AIDS in the Black community, the play tells the stories of a range of women with HIV, based on real-life interviews. Like the Pomos, Jones does not shy away from the socio-economic valences of the pandemic, homing in on concerns that disproportionately affect women with HIV. One of the young characters she channels, Stella, a young sex worker who states that she is 'dating' her father, exclaims: 'Sometimes I'd promise him the pussy, and I wouldn't even give him the pussy. We're not just born bitches! A lot of stuff happens to us. Now I got HIV. I mean WOW!!' (Jones 1998, 188). Another character, Nadine, seroconverts after years of heroin addiction linked to her abusive marriage. Meanwhile, Cookie reflects on the birth of her son, who is HIV-positive, telling him:

> Hey, come here. I love you, yes I do. I love you. Ofah … you getting so big. He was born premature. He weighed just two pounds. They didn't think he was going to make it! But here he is. Even with this HIV thing, I got a reason to live, I'm gonna be around for the cure. (Jones 1998, 188).

Clearly, Stella and Nadine experience their HIV diagnoses in ways deeply entwined with their subjugation as women attempting to survive capitalism's patriarchal structures, while Cookie introduces the audience to the biomedical concerns pregnant women experience.

Deep in the Night is very short, with a playtext spanning only fifteen pages. While it does not take such explicit aim at the individuals and structures responsible for the inequalities and prejudices shaping the pandemic, its unflinching approach to women's experiences serves to redress lacunae within the HIV/AIDS genre, confronting audiences with the pain and suffering that affected Black, HIV-positive women in the late 1990s. Like the Pomos, Jones is careful to thread a sense of political urgency through *Deep in the Night*, with the narrator stating: 'As the millennium approaches, in the midst of desire, disease, death and destruction, we pray for guidance. Oya! We rush to temple, to church.

On our knees we light candles. We chant. In this time of desperation, alienation and disaster we fitfully build altars' (Jones 1997, 184). The invocation of the phrase 'millennium approaches' – the title of the first part of *Angels in America* – establishes Jones's play within a wider canon of HIV/AIDS theater dominated by white men. In so doing, it encourages critical comparisons between *Deep in the Night* and more critically lauded and publicized plays, like those mentioned earlier in this book. As the fitful construction of altars attests, the women for whom Jones speaks are scrabbling for a coherent politics that suits their needs and demands – something playwrights like Kramer and Miller enjoy in their rallying cries against Republicans, evangelicals, and (for Kramer, at least) fellow members of the gay community. While there is hope (in Cookie's maternal relationship, for example), the question lingers as to how to address the various oppressions Jones's women face in combination with their HIV diagnosis. As it stands, the play's function is to garner empathy through outpourings of raw emotion and the laying bare of cruelties done toward its characters. As we will see, the prospects for developing a dissident, more cohesive politics remain tough in an increasingly neoliberal twenty-first century.

Black HIV/AIDS plays in the twenty-first century

As the twenty-first century drew near, caustic critique started to disappear from the stage. The Pomos disbanded in 1995, after which point HIV/AIDS theater shifted away from its more experimental and overtly political practices. At the same time as the introduction of potentially life-extending protease inhibitors legitimized the creation and revival of nostalgic plays, the ongoing neoliberalization of healthcare spawned a new generation of awareness-style theater that ultimately obscured governmental complicity in having allowed the crisis to intensify for over a decade. As we will see in the following chapter, neoliberalism's tendency to individualize responsibility for solving (or simply bearing) complex societal problems gave way to a raft of HIV/AIDS plays designed to equip spectators with knowledge about protecting themselves against infection.

While the HIV/AIDS genre has largely remained the domain of the white, gay, and moneyed in the twenty-first century, there have been some concerted attempts – albeit they have been relatively provincial – to explore the potential of theater to directly tackle sky-high infection rates within pockets of Black America. What I find most striking about the little scholarship that exists on Black HIV/AIDS theater is that much of it has emerged from social science disciplines and aims to quantifiably measure the extent to which plays can help reduce the spread of HIV. Take, for example, a study published by the *Journal of Black Sexuality and Relationships*, entitled 'The Exploration of Theater as an Innovative Tool to Improve HIV Rates Among Black Men' (2015), in which a group of researchers surveyed Black university students before they attended a show called *Lovely Words*. Noting in their introduction to the study that there is nothing 'peculiar' about Black men's sexual behavior that would leave them more vulnerable to HIV exposure, the researchers found that, by most measures, knowledge surrounding HIV transmission and prevention did not significantly increase among audience members after watching the play (Reed et al. 2015, 89–90). After reviewing previous scholarship about such prevention efforts among similar cohorts of young people, the authors explain that 'the literature indicated that many college students appeared to have difficulty translating this knowledge into consistent behaviors that may protect their health' (Reed et al. 2015, 78), concluding, therefore, that 'further examination of [theater's] effectiveness in addressing HIV/AIDS is warranted' (Reed et al. 2015, 84). What such analysis misses, of course, are the various material factors affecting how viruses spread within certain constituencies. In a country like the US – where access to quality healthcare is highly contingent on one's socio-economic status – knowledge alone is insufficient to quell infection rates.

Such pedagogical analysis also overlooks the potential for relatively recent medical innovations such as pre-exposure prophylaxis (PrEP) to ameliorate the problem. A safe and effective drug, PrEP can reduce an HIV-negative person's chances of seroconversion following sex or injection drug use. Despite its potential to transform the landscape of HIV/AIDS transmission, only 8% of Black people eligible for PrEP were prescribed the drug in the US in 2019 due to a constellation of limiting factors, including lack of access to healthcare, housing insecurity, stigma, and lack of access to transportation (Boerner 2022). For the most part, commercial awareness plays and the studies that emerge from them place the responsibility for tackling the epidemic on individuals, reiterating the importance of safe sex, while overlooking the material inequities and healthcare disparities that contribute to high rates of infection among Black gay and bisexual men. However well-intentioned the producers of such work, they ultimately buy into neoliberal forms of common sense that obscure the structural economic problems perpetuating the HIV/AIDS epidemic among poor and racialized constituencies.

Despite the dubious efficacy of safe sex awareness plays, the late 2010s and 2020s witnessed some increasingly politicized iterations of the genre. Take, for example, an immersive play called *As Much as I Can* (2017), directed by James Andrew Walsh and written by Sarah Hall. The play, which premiered in Baltimore in 2017 and hit New York's Public Theatre in 2019, represents a shift in the realm of mainstream HIV/AIDS theater. According to the show's publicity materials,

> If infection rates don't change, by 2020, 1 in 2 black men who have sex with men will be diagnosed with HIV in their lifetime. *As Much as I Can* (AMAIC) was created as a way to fight against this by empowering men to tell their own stories, fostering community dialogue, and reducing stigma. One of the first immersive theater productions that has been evaluated and demonstrated to be an effective public health intervention, AMAIC has toured the US regionally and premiered to sold out crowds in NYC with coverage from top tier press. In September 2019, AMAIC made its sold out Off-Broadway debut at the legendary Joe's Pub at the Public Theater. ('As Much as I Can' n.d.)

Upon entry to the show, audience members were assigned a color. Each color was associated with a different 'journey', as the play's writer terms it, taking groups of audience members to a range of settings, including a barbershop, a living room, a gay bar, a church, and a clinic. In each setting, actors recounted stories based on the real-life testimony of hundreds of men living with HIV, covering topics such as feelings of 'non-belonging', the relationship between diagnosis and drug use, homophobia in the Church, and what one actor describes as having 'an unhealthy relationship with going to the doctor' (Harley & Company 2019).

In many ways, the play marks an evolution in Black HIV/AIDS theater, opening up long-underexplored discussions about the relationship between race and HIV infection rates in America and drawing in rave reviews across the board, from *The New York Times* to *Teen Vogue*, thus spreading awareness of its central message beyond the strictures of the auditorium. Furthermore, its focus on stigma reveals an awareness of stigma's central role in perpetuating high infection rates. In so doing, the play represents a shift away from pedagogical work designed to impart knowledge about safe sex practices to its audience toward more community-minded oriented theater that, as one journalist put it, delivers 'passionate, truthful, and at times heartbreaking and intimate theatrical storytelling' (Sanchez 2019). The affective dimensions of *As Much as I Can* thus serve a political function in displacing prejudices surrounding HIV and cultivating greater empathy for those it affects – surely an important foundation on which to build a more solidaristic politics and encourage people who might have been exposed to HIV to seek care.

For all its novelty and capacity for building empathic bonds, however, the play skirts around the complex socio-economic dimensions of stigma and, therefore, overlooks the importance of challenging capitalism's role in perpetuating the spread of HIV. I do not wish to understate the play's role in raising awareness of HIV infection rates among young Black men in the US and imparting valuable knowledge to attendees, evidenced by the significant praise and press coverage garnered during its New York run. However, within the broader context of HIV/AIDS theater, the play's individualized approach and the lack of more dissident alternatives are symptomatic of a broader and enduring depoliticization of the genre. What *As Much as I Can* overestimates is the extent to which awareness of the importance of self-acceptance and employing de-stigmatizing language might act as a force for change. While stigma continues to play a major role in the failure to adequately address the HIV/AIDS crisis, the interactive form and content of the play presents stigma as an epiphenomenal pathology rather than what Tyler has designated as a form of power enmeshed within histories of capitalism, colonialism, and patriarchy.

Hall illustrates the cognitive behavioral logics undergirding the play in an interview about her writing process, explaining:

> I've studied a lot of neuroscience and cognitive science. As human beings, we act as though the social constructs that we create are unavoidable and absolute, and they are just things that we have all decided to participate in. And the minute that we decide not to participate in them, they are no longer true. So my work and this play is very much about saying, "We are so powerful, and that if we decide to believe in a different reality, we can have it tomorrow." It's also getting people to realize their power. (Berger 2019)

The idea that 'we have all decided to participate in' social constructs flattens the hierarchical and coercive aspects of hegemony that mold our collective reality, reflecting current discourse that 'brackets off from consideration the ways in which stigma is purposefully crafted as a strategy of government, in ways that often deliberately seek to foment and accentuate inequalities and injustices' (Tyler 2020, 18). As Gramsci emphasized, maintaining hegemony requires dominant powers to rule through coercive apparatuses that force compliance, as well as by manipulating the realm of common-sense ideas. Laying equal blame for societal ills at the feet of all ignores the ways in which state powers perpetuate stigma by enacting oppressive regulations and building a prejudicial consensus through rhetorical devices such as the 'welfare queen'. Thus, the play's politics are necessarily imbricated in neoliberal healthcare discourses of personal responsibility that view prejudicial attitudes as pathological and individually rectifiable, rather than serving a systemic role in the struggle for hegemony.

Beyond the play's rather thin analysis of prejudice, I would be remiss not to mention the role of its funding and advertising model in supporting a particular kind of capitalistic politics. *As Much as I Can* sells itself as a public health measure and received funding from GlaxoSmithKline's specialist HIV subsidiary, ViiV Healthcare (which also happens to be one of its most lucrative). As one public relations specialist noted in a press release reacting to the play, pharmaceutical companies could learn from ViiV Healthcare's project. The play, he claims, shows that the perspectives of those most affected by the virus should 'be central to the design of any care or support efforts', and that branded messaging

> should consider that care is for everyone, not just for people who are HIV+. And accessible, individual benefits—like getting or staying healthy—should be focused on instead of intangible, global goals, like ending the disease, which don't usually speak to people. Similarly, people should be offered care choices that are in line with their own ambitions and lifestyle preferences. All of these reflect a larger take-away: that a single patient population should never be spoken to as a homogenous group. (Abramowitz 2019)

Necessarily enmeshed in a system to which HIV/AIDS activists have traditionally been in opposition, the play cannot help but enter the PR machine of its benefactor, precluding or subduing commentary on the socio-economic causes of HIV spread and the deep injustices of America's healthcare system. As this public communications specialist helpfully spells out, pharmaceutical companies want us to dismiss as unrealistic the possibility of addressing the HIV/AIDS crisis at a global scale and from a universalist perspective, rationalizing this approach by pointing to the neoliberal subject's supposed lack of empathic capacities or inability to envisage the 'intangible' end of the pandemic. To make such an end tangible would, most likely, require us to think beyond capitalist modes of distribution, after all. To remain profitable and drive so-called 'innovation', pharmaceutical brands must focus on satisfying individuals' lifestyle preferences – hardly the communitarian approach we need to tackle material inequalities and stigma within all communities affected by HIV/AIDS.

To engage with a more radical, anti-capitalist politics would, obviously, contravene the profit-making principles on which pharmaceutical companies secure their long-term survival. Thus, projects like *As Much as I Can* obscure the reality of the HIV/AIDS crisis as systemic, allowing some of the follies of white nostalgic AIDS plays (i.e., their more sentimental and affective imperatives) to be repackaged and rigidified for profit-making ends. While the play undoubtedly goes some way to raising awareness about the significant problem of HIV/AIDS in communities of color, the promotional material surrounding the play clearly contains elements of Táíwò's aforementioned elite capture, cynically harnessing the tenets of standpoint epistemology to advocate for hyper-individualized forms of care that ignore the global scale of the crisis.

To wrap up this chapter, I turn to a recent play that takes a more experimental and confrontational approach to the politics of HIV/AIDS within Black communities, resisting some of the neoliberal imperatives to which contemporary playwrights are beholden. Donja R. Love's *one in two* (2019) is a short, semi-autobiographical play whose title alludes to the alarming statistic that half of all gay and bisexual Black men in the US will seroconvert at some point in their lives. First staged off-Broadway at the Pershing Square Signature Center, Love's play begins in what appears to be a white, sterile waiting room containing a large, floating number that gradually increases throughout the play – an ominous representation of the growing number of HIV/AIDS-related deaths in the US. At the same time, three topless Black men stand in a row, awaiting their fate. While such stagecraft clearly heralds a tale about HIV and its prevalence among queer Black men, the play starts with a seemingly unrelated metatheatrical game between the actors and the audience. Denoted in the playtext as Person on the Left, Person in the Middle, and Person on the Right, the men ask the audience to clap for one of them for no other reason than 'We're here because of them. So why not?' (Love 2022, 11). As it turns out, the selection system is designed to allocate roles for the rest of the play, with the person who receives the loudest applause assigned the ambiguous role of Number One. While the audience are given little clue as to the consequences of their choices, it quickly becomes clear that the role of Number One is less than desirable, as he resists the assignment and, after a little cajoling, concedes, 'Ugh! Fine. I'm Number One. Okay? Happy? Stop staring at me and figure out who's gonna be

Number Two and who will be Number Three between you two' (Love 2022, 13).

Having been assigned their roles, the men start with a flashback to their childhoods, playing a carefree game of duck-duck-goose. Soon, however, Number One grows frustrated with the scene and refuses to continue, looking at the rising number floating above the stage and stating, 'I'm not just a number' and 'We're done. If you're gonna keep us in here, we're gonna control what we do and how this shit go from now on. (*To The Numbers*). Not you!' (Love 2022, 15). In resisting his role and the gradual tick of the numbers, Number One critiques the power dynamics that exist between the audience and performers. He is not willing to present the stories they want to consume, geared as they are toward eventual doom and death, proceeding instead to tell a fragmented story of his HIV diagnosis and its attendant struggles, such as shame, alcoholism, and familial ignorance. The story is interspersed with further metatheatrical tussles and jests, as the men discuss the merits and perils of telling particular types of stories, while Number One – whose character we learn is called Donté – wonders whether to end Donté's life by suicide. Number Three resigns himself to an eventual tragedy, pointing at the audience and claiming, 'We're here because of them. They came to see a story. A story that has a beginning, a middle, and an END! An end to Donté's life. They like shit like that. Black Death gets through to them' (Love 2022, 50). Clearly, this statement and much of the play's audience engagement rests on its audience reflecting the largely white, middle-class constituencies that make up New York's theatergoing public – a virtually guaranteed scenario. For Number Three, the privileged audience appears only to consider the play's characters sympathetic in death – figures on which to project their liberal moralism without having to face up to the complex, contradictory, and sometimes unglamorous aspects of the men's lives. Thus, theatergoers can avoid thinking about the ways in which their material wealth and social standing contributes to wider societal inequalities and, by extension, their participation in a system that facilitates the characters' misery in the first place.

Number Two is unwilling to abide this audience–performer relationship, criticizing the very act of staging a play about HIV/AIDS in the absence of more solidaristic action to tackle the pandemic, implicating the audience in a kind of condescending and sinister voyeurism. He states: 'My story isn't important because I don't look like I could've been in *The Normal Heart* or *Angels in A-fucking-merica*? Is that it? Well… I just wish everyone would stop staring at me, stop "wishing me well" and do something. Anything' (Love 2022, 56). Like the Pomos, Love brings up theatrical touchstones of the HIV/AIDS crisis to shine a light on the genre's homogeneity and highlight the insidious nature of AIDS nostalgia. Rather than sit around watching the numbers rise, he implies, why are the supposedly justice-oriented audience not out on the streets fighting healthcare disparities? Of course, the very fact that Love and the play's wider crew bothered to stage *one in two* in the first place implicitly belies this pessimistic sentiment. Rather than denigrate the value of theater, the sustained metatheatrical probing of the audience members and their intentions serves to highlight the difficulties of staging work about HIV/AIDS in Black communities against the backdrop of a wider, strikingly homogeneous genre heavy with tired tropes and expectations. Less a play about HIV/AIDS itself than the experience of stigma and facing up to others' prejudices, Love's work antagonizes and discomfits spectators in a bid to shake up what have come to be the genre's most depoliticizing aspects – sentimentalism, sexual moralism, and inattention to the structural factors behind the spread of HIV/AIDS.

In critiquing the very genre of HIV/AIDS theater, Love intimates that addressing HIV/AIDS among some of society's most marginalized groups requires a significant shift in public consciousness. This sentiment aligns with Jih-Fei Cheng's belief that we cannot hope to build effective change across institutions such as universities and theaters without altering their terms of power. To address disparities in knowledge production, 'we cannot begin with AIDS as the object of study within our institutions or as the central object of critique in our social movements', lest women of color and queer and trans peoples of color become sidelined as afterthoughts to established (and exclusionary) narratives about AIDS (Cheng 2020, 77). Filtered through hegemonically aligned institutional structures, HIV/AIDS plays addressing underrepresented groups are subject to tokenistic treatment, molded around the requisites of a distinctly neoliberal form of identity politics that glosses over racial capitalism's structural inequities. While *one in two* does not directly critique capitalism, it recognizes the need for solidaristic politics as the foundation to significantly transform the lives of HIV-positive people across the US and beyond. Rather than subjects to be pitied or taught about safe sex practices, Love implies, marginalized groups deserve concrete, material assistance. This message is underlined at the end of the play, in which the stage directions prohibit any kind of curtain call: '*The play may seem over, but it's not. One in two Black gay men still receives an HIV diagnosis. Since The Numbers continue to grow, we have no reason to applaud. Until this statistic ends, there is no curtain call*' (Love 2022, 57). If the audience wants a satisfactory end to the play, they will need to work for it – to sacrifice some of their own comfort, time, or wealth to tackle the play's eponymous statistic.

Faced with the threat of elite capture and the continued veneration of whitewashed nostalgic plays, perhaps the solution for politicized playwrights interested in the racialized aspects of the epidemic in America lies in an explicit break from the HIV/AIDS genre and its history. As Love's play demonstrates, the theater sector and its audiences are fraught with preconceptions hostile to the development of plays capable of grasping the socio-economic foundations of the HIV/AIDS pandemic. Despite the play's diagnostic trenchancy, however, it leaves the audience to come up with solutions to the spread of HIV/AIDS in communities of color. So, what might a more action-oriented, counterhegemonic HIV/AIDS theater look like? As we will explore in the next chapter, the creation of activist or dissident work has become increasingly difficult as popular notions that the HIV/AIDS crisis is 'over' or solvable via neoliberal healthcare pedagogies proliferate. Indeed, HIV/AIDS plays have increasingly taken the form of monologic or documentary-style work, fashioned in such a way as to reduce transmission rates by individualizing responsibility and demonizing sexual subcultures. For theater or performance work to have any positive impact on marginalized communities struggling with HIV spread, we must further grapple with this trend.

CHAPTER FOUR

HIV/AIDS Theater as Public Health Measure

Although the HIV/AIDS theater genre has undergone a series of changes since its inception, by far the most significant has been its move toward more instrumentalist, public-health-oriented, and awareness-style performance modes. Following the introduction of a host of potentially life-prolonging antiretroviral drugs in the 1990s, including protease inhibitors, nucleoside reverse transcriptase inhibitors, and non-nucleoside reverse transcriptase inhibitors, the urgency and anger that roiled through works as esthetically and politically disparate as *The Normal Heart* and *The Law of Remains* started to dissipate. While the virus continued to wreak havoc among more marginalized and invisibilized communities in the Global North, the seemingly miraculous restoration of health among some members of wealthier populations (often referred to as the 'Lazarus Effect') marked an affective turning point for the middle-class gay men who had created some of the best-known HIV/AIDS plays in the Global North. As conservative HIV-positive commentator Andrew Sullivan noted in an article for *The New York Times* crassly titled 'When Plagues End', 'something profound has occurred these last few months. The power of the newest drugs [...] is such that a diagnosis of H.I.V. infection is not just different in degree today than, say, five years ago. It is different in kind. It no longer signifies death. It merely signifies illness' (Sullivan 1996). That is, of course, until you consider the significant proportion of the global citizenry (and, indeed, the American populace) who lack access to life-prolonging drugs. While Sullivan briefly acknowledges their continued plight, he characterizes AIDS as a 'natural calamity' and argues that the epidemic assuaged American homophobia, as 'acquiescence in gay-baiting and gay-bashing became, even in its strongholds, inappropriate at a moment of tragedy' (Sullivan 1996). While Sullivan's clear desire to depoliticize the epidemic and obscure how governmental inaction contributed to its catastrophic scale by no means reflects the broader attitudes of white gay America, its optimism neatly illustrates how wealth and privilege can shape one's willingness to comprehend and fight injustice.

With the prospect of their almost certain deaths extinguished, many of those with the financial and social means to stage HIV/AIDS plays in popular theaters shifted their attention away from lambasting the powerful individuals and systems responsible for inaction on the epidemic toward maximizing awareness of the drugs on offer and minimizing stigma surrounding HIV/AIDS. As we will see, many such plays emphasized the individual responsibility of gay and bisexual men to engage in safe sex practices and equip themselves with knowledge about the virus. Such plays were naturally tailored to a specific audience that excluded women and other marginalized groups, a trend very much in keeping with the ways in which governments, media organizations, and medical institutions treated these constituencies. As noted in Chapter 1, AIDS often presented differently in HIV-positive women, many of whom experienced symptoms such as pelvic inflammatory disease and irregular cervical smears. Consequently, women were often diagnosed at a much later stage than men and suffered worse outcomes as a result. Combined with the fact that 'social and economic conditions were dramatically different for many women with AIDS as compared to middle-class gay men', the government and media often overlooked the problem, meaning women were excluded from medical research and did not benefit from therapeutic assistance to the same extent as men (Schulman 2021a, 227). As many of the plays produced after the introduction of protease inhibitors were marketed as public health measures, they were typically structured around contemporary medical orthodoxies. Consequently, narratives typically centered on the lives of gay and bisexual men, compounding extant systemic erasures and inequities.

Asserting the monopoly white, gay, male populations have held over the production and shape of HIV/AIDS theater since the emergence of the AIDS crisis is not to place blame on individual theater makers. For the most part, creators of these cultural products appear to have acted in good faith, with the aim of improving the lives and health outcomes of audience members. Rather, by analyzing the broad trends that characterize the HIV/AIDS theater genre, we can uncover the systemic forces that have contributed to its (at least partial) depoliticization and subsumption into increasingly neoliberalized institutions. The homogeneous nature of much contemporary HIV/AIDS theater is significantly overdetermined, with a confluence of factors working together to push the genre toward more sanitized and depoliticized forms. Beyond the influence of the 'Lazarus Effect' and the structurally prejudicial pharmaceutical industrial complex, for example, the increasing marketization of theater and the consequent demise of experimentalism played a significant role in the development of HIV/AIDS theater.

The dwindling of funds and resources available to artists – particularly those willing to experiment with form and content – has helped foment a culture of deep skepticism toward the 'usefulness' of cultural production over, say, technical innovation or scientific discovery. As Caridad Svich notes, 'the emphasis on box-office receipts, entertainment "value", and "marketable content" has caused some artists to not only question their life's work, but to stop working altogether' (Svich 2002, 17). As such, there was a stark return to naturalism around the year 2000, as theaters and playwrights strived to produce the most marketable, easily consumable plays. Theater director Roberta Levitow strikes a similarly mournful note, locating the demise of avant-garde or experimental forms of theater around the time of Reagan's inauguration, when the craft of her theater-making contemporaries became less sustainable:

> Funding evaporated but we carried on performing. To surprisingly fewer and fewer of our peers. Where had all the young radicals gone? Into business or family maintenance, I'm sure. Meanwhile, our parents stayed the course, at those dull big theatres we abhorred. And those dull big theatres hired us to do our somewhat less radical work for them. (Levitow 2002, 28)

Again, a new economic common sense was pushing dramaturgs out of the sector, dampening the creativity and experimental verve of theater making and programming. I will dig deeper into the particularities and political economy of theater funding in the next chapter. For now, however, it is worth bearing in mind that this all-encompassing shift toward marketable theater incentivized the production of 'low-risk' plays that avoided challenging audiences with counter-hegemonic messaging or narratives that subverted the (neo)liberal philosophies inculcated throughout much of society. Exceptions and subversionary projects existed within this institutional landscape, of course. For the most part, though, marketization played a pivotal role in the development of HIV/AIDS theater, neutralizing and disavowing the politics of its earlier instantiations.

This chapter will analyze what such neutralization looked like. More specifically, it will clarify how neoliberal tenets surrounding individual autonomy and personal responsibility emerged as the primary structuring logics animating a significant chunk of HIV/AIDS plays in the twenty-first century. Given theater makers' decreased abilities to widely disseminate work capable of worrying at hegemonic common sense, it is perhaps unsurprising that many plays parroted the public health messaging of institutions themselves in thrall to neoliberalism's ideological tide. As Kane Race argues in *Pleasure Consuming Medicine: The Queer Politics of Drugs* (2009), the introduction of effective protease inhibitors effectively 'privatized' the experience of HIV. As the use of criminal provisions to prosecute those who passed on the virus proliferated around the world, the idea that sex came with shared, community-wide responsibilities was undermined, and HIV prevention became a matter of ensuring seropositive individuals took on sole responsibility for containing the virus, thus absolving the state of its preventative obligations. Meanwhile, caring community practices and volunteerism within queer communities became increasingly marginal, ensuring that the epidemic came to be seen 'as an aggregate of disparate individuals with viruses capable of being managed by these individuals, "in partnership" with doctors' (Race 2009, 116).

Unsurprisingly, this individualizing approach negatively affected racialized and otherwise marginalized groups while leaving wealthier constituencies more likely to benefit from neoliberal public health measures. As Tony Sandset explains in a study of recent HIV health campaigns, while messaging tends to be much more 'sex positive' and 'inclusive' than it was in the past – with much rhetoric committing to 'leaving no one behind' – the 'reliance on biomedical interventions as well as the highlighting of neoliberal ideals within HIV preventive campaigns might, in the long run, lead to the most vulnerable becoming left behind, increasing their vulnerability' (Sandset 2019, 659). In closely allying itself with this public health movement, therefore, HIV/AIDS theater has failed to address its largely homogeneous past.

The rise of HIV/AIDS documentary theater

One of the most significant ways in which HIV/AIDS theater makers adhered to the politically neutralizing demands of theatrical institutions after the turn of the millennium was via testimonial, verbatim, and documentary formats – that is, theater partly or wholly based on the experiences of real-life subjects. In tying their storylines to such source materials, many documentary theater makers have claimed to produce more authentic, objective, or non-partisan plays than those who create fictional narratives. In some ways, this has allowed HIV/AIDS theater makers to channel the voices of seropositive people while renouncing potential accusations of partiality. The collection of testimonials adopts the guise of sociological fieldwork, with audience members invited to make up their own minds about issues such as transmission rates and queer sexual practices. Although this dramaturgical strategy ostensibly shields playwrights from antagonistic and politically motivated accusations of hyperbole, identitarianism, or propagandism, close analysis might reveal some of the ways in which hegemonic common sense shapes documentary plays. Whose voices are spotlighted? Is there any editing or fictionalization involved? How are subjects treated and acknowledged beyond the confines of the stage? Addressing such questions will reveal how documentary plays operate in relation to the dominant culture, as well as their underlying political imperatives.

Take Peter Darney's *5 Guys Chillin'* (2016), for example. First staged in London at an intimate pub-cum-theater called the King's Head,[1] the play promises to deliver a socially progressive corrective to prejudicial mainstream narratives surrounding chemsex, a subcultural practice generally undertaken by gay and bisexual men involving group sex and the consumption of illegal substances (most notably crystal methamphetamine [crystal meth] and Gamma Hydroxybutyrate [GHB]). The discovery of chemsex by some of the UK's most popular mainstream media outlets triggered a kind of moral panic around the mid-2010s thanks to concerns surrounding the relatively high prevalence of HIV among men who have sex with men and the health risks associated with illegal substances such as meth. Despite there being no clear evidence that the practice had contributed to increased rates of HIV transmission, outlets including Vice Media, BBC News, the *Guardian*, and the *Evening Standard* were quick to assert this unfounded link following the release of a sensationalist documentary film entitled *Chemsex* in 2015 (Hakim 2015), with the *Observer* branding the subculture a 'Horror Story' haunted by the prospect of disease (Flynn 2020). Flimsy 'scientific' discourse and familiar homophobic tropes have

1 The theater has since changed homes, moving from a pub in Islington to a much larger, 200-seat conventional venue in the same area.

invariably accompanied this media coverage, with common themes emerging that suggest:

> most, if not all, gay men's engagement with chemsex is a form of self-harm rooted in internalised homophobia and the resulting inability to form meaningful relationships with other gay men. That chemsex frequently leads to physical and mental health issues and sometimes death. That chemsex is linked to the recent increase in HIV transmission in the UK and therefore poses a public health crisis. (Hakim 2015)

Recognizing the need for a queer perspective on the topic and a corrective to the demonization of chemsex participants, Darney's play embarks on the politically and socially worthy mission to educate audiences about the mental and physical health issues associated with chemsex in a measured and non-pathologizing fashion. Based on the verbatim testimony of participants, the play tells a fictional story of a single chemsex party (or 'chill-out', to use the parlance of the subculture). Its characters – who are loosely based on Darney's real-life participants and referred to only by their initials (J, M, B, R, and PJ) – speak frankly about their experiences of the chemsex scene, swapping stories and exchanging words of advice in a way that, as detected by David Stuart in a foreword to the published text of the play, characterizes chemsex and its attendant risks as 'a community issue, one that will require compassion, unity, and the setting aside of our judgments and unkindness' (Stuart 2016, 14).

The impulse to construct counternarratives to mainstream media headlines has commonly been cited as a motivating factor in the creation of documentary theater in the UK. Popular examples include Robin Soans's *Talking to Terrorists* (2005), which sought to uncover the reasons why people commit terrorist atrocities via the verbatim testimony of perpetrators and, therefore, better convey the complexities of the so-called 'war on terror'. Soans's play, like others of its time, is the product of a political environment characterized by degradation of public faith in the integrity of institutions traditionally upheld as authoritative purveyors of truth, such as public service broadcasters. Locating the origins of this trend around the turn of the millennium, Daniel Schulze argues that spectators and audiences felt they were not being told the truth by public institutions in this era. Theater, for some, effectively took over the role of journalism, purporting to show the gritty reality behind official stories (Schulze 2017, 193).

While this conception of documentary theater as a uniquely dependable form of knowledge has clearly proved compelling, scholars have been quick to point out the folly in uncritically accepting its truth-telling function. As Stephen Bottoms notes, the apparent realism of the verbatim form 'purports to present a transparent representation of "lifelike" behaviour, while in fact providing a constructed authorial perspective on the real', which conflates editorial creativity with incontrovertible authority over truth (Bottoms 2006, 59). The very structure of *Talking to Terrorists*, for example, in which a psychologist provides running analyses and diagnoses for its interviewees, betrays Soans's desire to 'other' and pathologize his subjects from the outset. The psychologist's '"insights" function to circumvent any need for actual comprehension of the possible motives behind political violence: we are assured that terrorists are simply dysfunctional unfortunates more to be pitied than feared' (Bottoms 2006, 58). By essentializing terrorists as somehow 'broken' or 'damaged' anomalies in this way, the play delegitimizes the complex political grievances that might have contributed to their violent actions: they become exemplars of the human capacity for evil while the state remains its innocent victim. Rather than deliver a counterhegemonic narrative that questions prevailing power structures, Soans's play cements their dominance and reveals how the documentary form remains acutely vulnerable to editorial bias and normative modes of thinking.

So, to what extent does *5 Guys Chillin'* achieve the measured narrative to which it stakes a claim? On the one hand, the fact we hear about real subjects' experiences, including their more light-hearted and amusing anecdotes concerning sexual mishaps and miscommunications, serves to humanize chemsex participants. As reviewer David Ralf notes,

> the loose conceit that these conversations are taking place at an actual party, and therefore are spoken to an audience of exclusively gay men – is a highlight, and these cheeky, happy moments are both what distinguish the play from the reporting about chemsex, and are key to learning about a subculture that is so fraught with sensationalist bad news. (Ralf 2016)

However, despite well-meaning intentions to undermine the demonization of chemsex participants, Darney's play slips into common-sense modes of thought in a similar way to Soans's, peddling neoliberal tenets that apotheosize 'wellbeing', self-reliance, monogamy, and ostensibly 'healthy' lifestyle habits. Readers are probably acutely aware of the ways in which 'wellbeing' discourse has proliferated in line with neoliberalism's growing stranglehold on society. As decades of financialization and deregulation have eroded real wages and living standards for all but the very few, mental health issues such as anxiety and depression have grown in kind. By extension, organizations and institutions of various types have relied on 'wellbeing' initiatives to quell political malaise and shore up psychic investment in neoliberal structures. As is capital's wont, corporate powers and state functionaries maximize private gains and minimize public spending by promoting activities such as 'self-care', yoga, journaling, and other (cheap) metaphorical sticking plasters, while failing to distribute the material wealth and resources that could help build a happier and healthier society.

What renders documentary theater such a fertile form through which to peddle this neoliberal wellbeing ethic is its appeal to authenticity. To elucidate how, I turn to Roger Foster's short essay, 'Therapeutic Culture, Authenticity, and Neoliberalism', which argues that the concept of authenticity – or, at least, the ability to 'live authentically' and follow one's 'true passions' – has become a normative indicator of happiness, health, and success (Foster 2016, 101). Although the possibility of embracing a kind of 'true self' untouched by society's influences and pressures is quite clearly illusory, its rhetorical appeal to personal autonomy is highly seductive in a neoliberal context. In a system prioritizing surplus value extraction and growth above all else, the personal and democratic freedoms afforded to those who create such value are necessarily circumscribed. Stripped of many social democratic freedoms, welfare provisions, and other public goods, the neoliberal subject's agential powers are largely confined to the sphere of consumer culture (Gilbert and Williams 2022, 117). Within the logical confines of this sphere, freedom's notoriously inchoate essence starts to crystallize as the ability to express oneself through personal consumption – in other words, the clothes one buys and the hobbies one adopts.

To elucidate how this phenomenon contributed to the formation of contemporary health and wellness culture, Foster returns to Herbert Marcuse's theories surrounding scientism and technological rationality, applying them to a neoliberal context by analyzing how contemporary therapeutic disciplines such as psychology often encourage us to conceptualize individual autonomy in paradoxically oppressive and instrumental terms. Conceived during the increasingly consumerist 1960s, Marcuse's *One-Dimensional Man* (1964) argued that improvements in material living standards initially brought about by advanced industrial capitalism obfuscated the antagonistic social relations that constitute class struggle in a classically Marxian sense. To shore up hegemonic consensus yet further, new forms of consumerist advertising and mass media were enlisted to perpetuate teleological narratives of technological progress:

> Within the vast hierarchy of executive and managerial boards extending far beyond the individual establishment into scientific laboratory and research institute, the national government and national purpose, the tangible source of exploitation disappears behind the façade of objective rationality. Hatred and frustration are deprived of their specific target, and the technological veil conceals the reproduction of inequality and enslavement. (Marcuse [1964] 2002, 35)

Foster argues that such forms of control have only intensified and broadened into new areas in a neoliberal context, as ostensibly objective or 'commonsensical' psychological maxims surrounding authenticity and wellness smother the counterhegemonic potential of neoliberal subjects, numbing the discomfort and burnout engendered by neoliberalism's imperative to produce.

Although the twenty-first century has witnessed increasing social inequality and disunity thanks to the relentless financialization of the economy and other neoliberal phenomena, the dominant culture attempts to obfuscate this problem by popularizing individualized psychotherapy and self-help methodologies. The goal, it seems, is to help governments enact oppressive and immiserating policies on their citizenries with relatively little backlash. As Foster explains, this hegemonic shift was achieved by the increased standing of professional expertise in 'what [Nikolas Rose] calls the "psy" disciplines, such as psychology and psychiatry'. Given that 'liberal conceptions of government generally forbid the direct action of the state upon individual life-plans and choices, government must act in an indirect manner upon the wishes, desires and values of subjects' (Foster 2016, 105). Contemporary therapeutic culture, which places considerable value on the so-called 'psy' disciplines and encourages the discovery of an essential, authentic self, thus provides 'individuals with the linguistic and cultural resources to make sense of their lives as the result of a series of choices, thus making individual lives amenable to new forms of intervention and management' (Foster 2016, 106). Decisions and actions that lie outside of this model – a model Foster terms the 'ethic of authenticity' – are, therefore, figured as deviant, immoral, or pathological. In many ways, the men depicted in *5GC* are shown to fail at the requisite self-monitoring required by therapeutic neoliberal governance, subverting or defying it in a way that is figured as harmful and in contravention of civic duty.

A scene toward the end of the play – and, indeed, the end of the 'chill-out' – exemplifies these apparent failings when a light-hearted interchange about sexual exploits is quickly disrupted by dark events. After listening to sexual anecdotes from PJ, M, and R about sleeping with colleagues, having sex while listening to the soundtracks of children's films, and enjoying the feeling of 'loads … squirting out of ass cheeks as you're walking down the road', B explains:

> B: (*They laugh.*) Yeh! I've, I've left the Hoist before now with an ass full of cum. And it's been leaking out while I've been walking home… I've been collecting it and eating it as I've been walking down the street! It must look so wrong. But I'm a cum addict…
>
> *Movement transition: R changes the music. Goddess by Chrome Spark. It moves to lust/sex. Just as M is about to fuck PJ, he G's out. They turn the music off – lighting snaps with it to a colder/bluer state. PJ's screams/fit continues for a moment in the stark silence as they hold him down. They put him in the recovery position, and he spends the rest of the play unconscious in the space. The mood is now darker/pensive/reflective. It's that moment when everyone has realised they should have got their Uber home an hour ago and they are too fucked to leave.* (Darney 2016, 48)

B's anecdote is the last in a series of humorous tales of increasingly illicit acts. Up to this point, the stories have not been imbued with any particularly moralistic messages, despite their traditionally abject nature. Indeed, the comic one-upmanship that appears to drive the interchange, with the men competing to offer as subversive anecdotes as possible, could be seen as intended to teasingly scandalize and provoke audience members who are not *au fait* with the subculture. However, the jarring shift in tone during the 'movement transition' casts a new meaning over the exchange and everything that came before it. PJ 'G's out', effectively overdosing on GHB, an industrial solvent often used recreationally during chemsex parties to generate feelings of confidence, sexual arousal, and euphoria. PJ's reaction to the drug appears to jolt the atmosphere of the party from something ecstatic and upbeat to something much more sinister, a shift reflected in the lighting and effects set out in the stage directions. By cutting out the music and bathing the stage in a cold, blue light, PJ's overdose is signified as a disruptive spectacle; a new phase in the evening's trajectory.

In this way, the audience is encouraged to reevaluate and question everything that occurred in the run-up to the event. PJ's loss of somatic control, for example, is emblematic of his inability to fulfill the imperative of responsibility for the self. He moves from a good-humored, active member of the group to one whose mental stability and even dignity are scrutinized. Certainly, the semiotics of PJ's body lying prostrate in the recovery position for the rest of the play operate as a constant reminder of the physical risks that inhere in certain chemsex practices and preclude any possibility of the party returning to its formerly spirited atmosphere. On the stage, an unmoving body could just as plausibly represent a dead person as an unconscious one, and the fact that the conscious men continue talking among themselves while ignoring PJ's body, with B and J even having sex next to PJ before the play ends, depicts a culture of pathological self-interest and anti-communitarianism that, if we recall the fictionalized nature of these events, contradicts documentary theater's claims toward journalistic neutrality. Rather than offering an alternative to mainstream narratives surrounding chemsex subculture, this scene compounds some of the widely disseminated criticisms commonly directed at its participants.

If the overdose scene were not sensationalist enough to scandalize an audience attuned to recent discussions surrounding chemsex, the play's final stage directions might well be:

> *B and J have sex on the floor next to unconscious PJ. R does a line. Smokes. Cries. He has not noticed the line of blood from his nose. Music swells. House-lights up – no curtain call. The party keeps going till the house is clear. The sense is that it will go on for days.* (Darney 2016, 54–5)

5GC culminates in an atmosphere of chaos, with R's bloody nose potentially reminding the audience of the seropositivity of his blood or, perhaps, a lack of self-care and compassion. The idea that the party will go on for days reinforces the idea that chemsex traps men in a cycle of self-destruction and plunders their so-called 'free will'. While I am wary of underplaying some of the well-documented and life-altering problems that chemsex can cause for its participants, it is safe to assert that the sensationalism of *5GC* contradicts any claims toward measured, panic-free discourse. If the play were to sincerely craft an 'authentic' portrayal of chemsex subculture, it would surely pay heed to some of the communitarian aspects that go beyond societal problems caused by individualistic pleasure seeking.

Writing about the intimate and troubled relationship between chemsex and HIV transmission, for example, Race claims that analyzing chemsex through a queer lens grounded in participants' experiences might provide a more incisive theory of HIV prevention. While chemsex spaces are often demonized as pathogenic by epidemiologists, these spaces are 'also key sites for the elaboration of significant social relationships and bonds. In these spaces, participants may be undertaking some of the affective groundwork that generates new possibilities of care, connection, relationality and transformation' (Race 2017, 134). Certainly, Darney's characters demonstrate little of this type of bonding. While partners B and R (who are involved in a three-person relationship) exchange affectionate words and comfort each other when faced with painful memories, any mention or performance of sexual acts that deviate from the tenets of traditional monogamy (or at least long-term commitment) serve only to disrupt this affective attachment. R in particular is figured as a victim of his partner's sexual brio and fervor, expressing a strong preference for the 'more intimate side of a relationship, like hugging and cuddling. The most fun about our relationship is when the three of us are lying in bed, watching a DVD. That's better than having twenty guys come and fuck around!' (Darney 2016, 54). In this brief penultimate line of *5GC*, its moralistic messaging is made clear: meaningful human connection may only be found within the confines of a (mostly) sexually exclusive union.

Other forms of sexual connection represent a failure of self-control or discipline and are invariably haunted by the negative prospects of HIV infection, drug dependency, overdose, and jealousy. It is in this way that the play reflects what Marcuse, building on a Freudian view of sublimation, conceives as one-dimensional society's tendency to steer instinctual erotic energies and social antagonisms into controlled modes of thought:

> Just as this society tends to reduce, and even absorb opposition [...] in the realm of politics and higher culture, so it does in the instinctual sphere. The result is the atrophy of the mental organs for grasping the contradictions and alternatives and, in the one remaining dimension of technological rationality, the *Happy Consciousness* comes to prevail. (Marcuse [1964] 2002, 82)

While Darney figures *5GC* as offering an alternative narrative to that popularized by the mainstream media, therefore, its focus on preserving a socially prized *Happy Consciousness* through a sexual schema in control of errant, destructive drives merely reinforces restrictive one-dimensionality.

In some ways, Darney's decision to anonymize his subjects equips him with the authorial license he needs to conduct neoliberalism's hegemonic work. While anonymization shows necessary deference to the ethical sensitivities bound up with using subjects' word-for-word experiences – vulnerable as they are to misrepresentation – it also provides Darney with a considerable amount of leeway to imbue the play with tacit ideological messages. Thanks to the degree of artistic license required to depict a party that never actually took place, it is virtually impossible to tell which parts of the text have been lifted verbatim and which are imagined. Thus, Darney is freed to some extent from the responsibility of fashioning characters faithful to the personalities and temperaments of the people on whom they are based, allowing him to pass off as fact moralistic speculations surrounding the ways in which chemsex culture negatively affects the lives of participants.

If there were any doubt as to the editorialization of *5GC*, the paratextual elements of its playtext should be proof enough. Although the 'Author's Note' stresses the importance of respecting the 'choice' and 'free will' of those who partake in chemsex, Darney also cites his inspiration for writing the play as a fascination with the 'buried sadness' he supposedly detected in a subject named J, as well as J's 'need for someone special to connect to' and his 'nihilistic tendencies' (Darney 2016, 1). Of course, the idea of 'buried' sadness is necessarily speculative in this context, indicating that Darney predetermined the story he had hoped to disinter before conducting research for the play.

Although David Stuart argues that '[b]ringing ChemSex to the stage … not only raises awareness of this difficult cultural phenomenon, but provides a safe space for the issues to be presented, explored, humanised; extricated from the scandal-mongering headlines that alarm and stigmatise the issue' (Stuart 2016, 13), the affective language Darney employs suggests that the play is more ideologically coercive than Stuart grasps. While *5GC*'s subjects are not demonized in the same way as chemsex participants are in many mainstream media outlets, they are figured as 'victims' in a way that sensationalizes chemsex subculture, pathologizing participants and thereby justifying its stigmatization. Perhaps most tellingly, the 'Author's Note' also explains how

> J came to see *5 Guys Chillin'* at the King's Head in its last run. He had been clean for forty-three days. I massively regret letting him come. The stress of being faced with that part of his life, in the company of his old chill mates, wasn't something he was ready for, and he relapsed. (Darney 2016, 8)

The use of the word 'letting' here suggests dominion over J and betrays an imagined managerial relationship with the subject. From the outset, therefore, it is clear Darney claims a monopoly over 'truth' in a similar way to Soans in *Talking to Terrorists*. He adopts a paternalistic role, condemning chemsex and dictating what he believes is best for those who participate. Furthermore, in subordinating J and asserting that his 'ability to choose with free will had gone', Darney declares, rather simplistically, that J faces a dichotomous choice between possessing the 'free will' to live 'authentically' or relinquishing all free will to the culture of chemsex (Darney 2016, 20). Such binarism exemplifies the neoliberal fashioning of self-management and responsibility as the common sense of a society in which, as Foster argues, the narrative of authenticity has collapsed 'into a therapeutic narrative of instrumental self-management' (Foster 2016, 111).

Having established the journalistic angle that runs throughout *5GC*, I return to the ways in which its sensationalist edge is undergirded by the therapeutic culture Foster links to neoliberal ideology. The distinctly therapeutic tone evident within much of the discourse preceding PJ's overdose is strongly indicative of a play that sanctions an 'ethic of authenticity', emulating the discourse of group therapy. The men share their thoughts, experiences, and secrets surrounding their chemsex habits, opening up opportunities for other characters to offer relevant thoughts and advice. Take, for example, a scene in which the men discuss issues surrounding sexual health after J recounts how he became HIV-positive:

> PJ: My wife's six months pregnant. (*Group is stunned.*) Scary. But I think being a parent saved my life in many ways… You know, I used to risk my life a lot. With unprotected sex. And I think – it made me love myself more. Changed the focus. Made me less selfish.
>
> R: I'm HIV positive too. I would not have bareback sex with a guy who said to me he was negative. If he turned round and said to me I'm negative, but I want to have sex bareback, I wouldn't believe him he could've had a test, what twelve weeks ago? And then caught HIV within that time, you know what I mean? So! When we play we play with other HIV guys.
>
> B: I'll play with negative guys!
>
> R: Errrrr!

J: You do have a responsibility to make sure that everybody else is safe. (Darney 2016, 43)

On one level, this passage demonstrates the subjects' adherence to (or at least acknowledgment of) safe sex practices designed to protect fellow participants in chemsex subculture, with the confessional mode acting as a measure of their 'authentic' commitment to communitarian harm reduction. However, pay close attention to the linguistic construction of the characters' divulgences and it becomes clear that a neoliberal social order shapes the experiences of these men. The self-referential nature of their discourse (they speak of others but only in relation to themselves) is illustrative of a distinctly neoliberal form of authenticity which 'rather than representing a tension between society and the individual [...] now works to foster social cohesion through its normalizing of the notions of individual responsibility and self-reliance' (Foster 2016, 108). J's assertion that a generalized 'you' has a responsibility toward 'everybody else', for example, is indicative of neoliberalism's ideological imperative to outsource or privatize health and social care into the hands of individuals. The problematic aspects of drug use as dangerous to physical and mental health are not the concern of state institutions and wider society but must be handled by the men alone.

This individualistic messaging is also consistent with a self-serving dialectic that allows men such as PJ to conceptualize procreation with his wife as a path toward self-betterment or 'self-love' (despite earlier confessing that he married to please his parents and extended family). As Foster explains, the contemporary neoliberal conception of authenticity is supported by self-help discourse embodying 'a therapeutic ethos that hides real economic and social failure and disappointment behind a projected fantasy of individual self-reliance through careful emotional management' (Foster 2016, 111). The ideal of self-reliance promulgated by *5GC*, then, refuses to place any responsibility for the safety of chemsex participants onto public institutions, thereby upholding neoliberal hegemony's mission to privatize social welfare. To give *5GC* its political dues for a moment, one could argue that the play critically interrogates PJ's self-betterment fantasy as an indictment of societal homophobia. His engagement with a practice that leaves him unconscious on a stranger's floor could easily be read as a destructive coping mechanism for dealing with life in a legally binding heterosexual union, for example.

However, the therapeutic processes and patterns that undergird the men's revelations are ultimately conceptualized as palliative when it comes to assuaging the 'buried sadness' Darney identifies in J and, by extension, the other partygoers. There are clearly identifiable patterns in the play's oscillation between moments of 'authentic' confessional discourse and those in which sexual acts and drug taking occur: therapeutic revelations are followed by further affective disclosures, hugging and platonic affection, while sexual acts tend to be followed by tension, conflict or, in the case of PJ, a loss of somatic control. In this way, the play can be seen to advocate the kind of robust emotional management facilitated by therapeutic sessions, while drug taking and sex (the core activities that constitute chemsex and bring the men together in the first place) are figured as antithetical to this aim.

While PJ's revelations might throw up a wide range of ethical issues, other partygoers markedly forgo the opportunity to explore them, choosing (as does R) to swiftly move on to stories of their own. In so doing, they refuse to problematize or interrogate PJ's apparent self-love in such a way that betrays possible capitulation to something Lee Edelman (in)famously termed 'reproductive futurism', an unwavering belief in the generalized Child as the figure for whose benefit political and moral decisions should be made. Such a belief necessarily restricts the scope of political discourse and secures 'the absolute privilege of heteronormativity by rendering unthinkable, by casting outside the political domain, the possibility of a queer resistance to this organizing principle of communal relations' (Edelman 2004, 2). PJ's drive for self-preservation is framed according to his responsibility to stay fit and healthy for his children, while the politics of a heterosexual union he was effectively coerced into go virtually unproblematized. This reproductive futurism is underlined in the final scene, when the self-governance for which PJ strives is shown to be lacking. Darney's editorial decision to have PJ – the party's only father – overdose, for example, draws particular attention to his failures of responsibility and self-control. The apparent indignity of lying prostrate on a gloomy stage serves as a warning against chemsex's potential to lure men away from their 'authentic selves' and, by extension, fail their loved ones and dependents.

PJ's responsibility to his offspring and the play's overriding message surrounding safe sex and individual responsibility are tightly imbricated throughout the play: if the content of *5GC* were not enough to remind audiences of its pedagogical aims, the fact that each audience member at the King's Head production received a free condom before the show (Hochstrasser 2017) surely makes clear the play's attachment to neoliberal notions of governance and personal responsibility. The rather one-sided ideological dimensions of Darney's documentary style did not go unnoticed in the press. Reviewer Paul Cockburn, for example, commented, 'for all its fun and darkness, *5 Guys Chillin'* feels like a well-meaning "safer sex" campaign' (Cockburn 2017). Gareth K. Vile is similarly conscious of this one-dimensionality:

> By the finale, when the darkest confessions emerge, the production has made its point. A generation of men are unable to have stable relationships, are carelessly catching STDs and damaging their bodies through an almost thoughtful desire for drugs and sex. It is as shocking as a government funded advert from the 1980s, with a tombstone casting a shadow over the cheeky, fun-seeking characters. (Vile 2016)

Vile is unequivocal about the didacticism of the play's message, invoking the UK government's controversial 'Don't Die of Ignorance' campaign to emphasize its potential to engender fear and panic in its audience.[2] The fact that *5GC* appears to him to indict a whole 'generation' of men is indicative of the journalistic sensationalism that, in many ways, this study identifies as the primary failing of much discourse surrounding chemsex. If writers of documentary theater are to get anywhere near the realms of truth, ethical representation, or indeed authenticity (with all of the problems and ambiguities these things entail), they must explore the necessarily imperfect nature of the very form they adopt.

As Bottoms notes, documentary plays that are aware of their own constructedness 'encourage spectators to think for themselves about the process of representation involved' in portraying reality, and adopt a more critical, multidimensional approach to spectatorship (Bottoms 2006, 67). Thanks to its reliance on spectacle and one-track claims toward a solution to 'fix' the issues surrounding the chemsex scene, *5GC* forecloses such an opportunity. Darney uses the documentary form to achieve a kind of authenticity that is vitiated by neoliberal ideology as a technology of dominance and control. To this extent, *5GC* unveils just some of the ideological traps to which documentary theater is vulnerable in the contexts of public health and harm reduction strategies.

2 As part of the campaign, the government released an advert featuring ominous music and a tombstone emblazoned with the word 'AIDS'. The advert finishes with the warning: 'If you ignore AIDS, it could be the death of you' (Central Office of Information for Department of Health 1987)

Experimental dramaturgies and public health messaging

While documentary and testimonial forms represent mainstays of public-health-focused theater, some HIV/AIDS playwrights have employed more experimental, fictionalized dramaturgies to address the changing landscape of HIV/AIDS prevention and management. One of the most significant disruptive forces to have altered the lives of HIV-positive gay men since the beginning of the millennium is the indomitable rise of Web 2.0. Having precipitated the rise of dating and hookup apps, as well as other forms of online sociality, digital culture has altered the spaces through which status disclosure and discussions surrounding HIV take place. For example, online serosorting, or the practice of seeking out sexual partners of the same HIV status in order to minimize the transmission risk, has emerged as an alternative sexual health measure to those sanctioned by public health bodies and the medical establishment.

The political implications of apps such as Grindr represent a contentious point of discussion in queer academic circles. As Tim Dean explains in one of the most widely cited works on bareback sex, *Unlimited Intimacy: Reflections on the Subculture of Barebacking* (2009), bareback cruising in the pre-Grindr era arguably reflected an ethos of caring and hospitality toward strangers that serves to critique the individualistic rhetoric often associated with healthcare institutions promoting safe sex. Today, however, the vast proportion of bareback sex is negotiated online, 'where the attitude of openness threatens to deteriorate into a controlled instrumentalization of the other as an object of use' (Dean 2009, 194). This notion that dating apps dehumanize participants, presenting them as an assemblage of essentially fungible attributes (including HIV status), is a criticism frequently directed toward such platforms, regardless of whether they cater for straight or queer communities.

However, as Tom Roach counters in an essay on queer intimacies in social media, the dehumanizing aspects of apps such as Grindr can actually feed their uptake, reflecting a form of individualism purely driven by the pursuit of pleasure and destruction of the ego that might violate such a neoliberal paradigm. While anti-neoliberal critiques offer up rational grievances when it comes to instrumentalization, the apparent 'nonsense' of online cruising must be adequately probed to discover what Roach figures as the ambivalence at its heart; that is, the elements of online cruising that seek out 'alternative presents, other futures' (Roach 2015, 78). While the impersonal elements of online hookups might encourage a mercenary attitude toward relationship building and HIV transmission control, 'we might [also] understand online MSM [men who have sex with men] cruising as a contemporary site in which a queer ethics [...] seeks to outgrow the present, outlive sexuality, and outsmart, or, perhaps, "outdumb," the maneuverings of liberal rationality' (Roach 2015, 78). In other words, the online cruising space might represent somewhere that can transcend neoliberal health rationalities by facilitating interactions unshackled from a kind of *quid pro quo* logic toward an ethics of care and prosociality.

Perhaps unsurprisingly, many HIV/AIDS playwrights have produced work that intervenes in debates about how apps like Grindr affect the lives of seropositive people. Take Lachlan Philpott's *Bison* (2009), for example, which employs experimental dramaturgical techniques to mimic aspects of digital discourse and critique the contemporary gay scene. The play starts with a scene set in what, we soon infer, is a waiting room of men getting tested for HIV. The characters are not named, and are denoted in the playtext simply as 1, 2, 3, and 4. As illustrated by the following extract, they narrate a detailed account of their non-verbal communications while tension surrounding their impending test results seems to saturate the room:

1 Eyes in this room with nowhere to rest. Get it out of the way.
1–4 Clock ticks
2 He's looking at me/
3 He's looking away/
4 I'm looking at him/
1 I'm looking away
3 him behind the frosted window/
2 his lips/
1 mouths words, asks something
4 smutty fuck me grin/hey
2/3 Hey
4/1 hey/
3 clock ticks
2 door opens/
4 door shuts/
...
1–4 Clock ticks.
1 I'm 32/
2 I'm 17
4 I'm 29/

3 45, 46, 47, 48
2 Am I too late?
3 Am I too late?
1–4 am I too late? (Philpott 2010, 26–7)

The body is used as the primary means of interaction in the waiting room, as characters employ gesture and non-linguistic communication while awaiting their results. The flirtatious games played with characters' eyes, the visual language saturating the 'smutty fuck me grin', and the way in which a character's lips metonymically 'mouths words' combine to suggest a carnality to these relationships that transcends the need for verbal communication. The scene also illustrates an intense focus on temporality with the repeated chorus of 'clock ticks' and the urgent refrain of 'am I too late?', both of which intimate that they are on course for premature death and, therefore, trapped in the era preceding the introduction of protease inhibitors.

While the virus is, of course, a tragic harbinger, it also represents an impetus for bonding and communitarianism as the men use their collective fate as an excuse to play flirtatious games. That they share their ages with their peers and the audience before the final chorus of 'am I too late' not only emphasizes the tragedy of diagnosis but allows the men to share in each other's pain and look beyond their immediate personal interests. While there is no explicit mention of HIV/AIDS, the brevity of this scene (in the playtext it spans only two pages), combined with the fact that the characters are unnamed and inhabiting an ambiguous spatio-temporality, encourages audience members to find connections or points of difference between this inaugural exchange and later scenes set in the twenty-first century.

Take, for example, the following exchange representing discussion on an online hookup forum, in which HIV has become one of many 'stats' involved in sexual negotiation:

1 inked?/
4 pierced?/
1 hung?/
1–4 horny?
1 poz?
2 neg?
1 poz?
4 neg?
1/2/4 disease free?...
2 swimmer's build

4 labourer's build
2 diver's build. (Philpott 2010, 35)

This passage aligns with Race's conception of the online user profile as a 'market device' that 'equips users with certain capacities and formats practices of self-representation, informing activities such as searching, evaluating, sorting and selecting among the various "goods" on offer' (Race 2017, 54). The positioning of the questions 'neg?' and 'poz?' alongside requests for information about relatively superficial physical attributes such as whether interlocutors are tattooed, or the size of their genitals, appears to illustrate the commodification (and, indeed, fetishization) of HIV. Abbreviating 'positive' and 'negative' to the slangy 'poz' and 'neg' dilutes the complex political and affective dimensions of HIV status disclosure, downgrading the virus to just one of myriad sexual preferences in an online marketplace. At the same time, the staccato rhythm and almost stichomythic interchange of the above passage demonstrates the reduction of safe sex negotiation to something akin to an auction or stock exchange, situating it somewhere in the realm of commerce. In this way, *Bison* tracks the shifting dynamics of sexual negotiation as it moves ever further into the digital domain, the consequences of which warrant scrutiny when examining topics such as serosorting.

As mentioned earlier, Tim Dean argues against the instrumentalizing function of platforms such as Grindr, particularly when it comes to online serosorting, claiming that it goes against the communitarian, nurturing, and anti-establishment ethos afforded by other kinds of virus containment practices. This argument is compelling insofar as the promotional and self-seeking imperatives of any online platform reflect wider attitudes that are integral to the so-called free market. However, while the strong influence of neoliberal self-interest on digital hookup media is quite clear, online forums retain kernels of counterhegemonic power that complicate Dean's critique. Roach, for example, defends the 'ego-lessening indignities and pleasures' generated by such cold and pragmatic exchanges (Roach 2015, 60). Despite its potentially alienating function, the online interface might help nurture affective bonds, as 'in the virtual atmosphere of shared estrangement, the destructive ego might be humbled if not humiliated, unknown selves and unusual intimacies born, and respect for the inviolable alterity of the other learned' (Roach 2015, 57).

Following Leo Bersani's ideas surrounding cruising as constitutive of a 'scattering' of the self among superficial acquaintances, or akin to 'ecological' rhythms like the cycle of the moon, Roach believes the online forum facilitates a 'flittering among aestheticized object-others [that] moves to a music that exceeds the ebb and flow of individualized desire' (Roach 2015, 67). Using the popular hookup app Grindr as an exemplary instrument of the aforementioned self-scattering, for example, Roach compares the appearance of its gridded interface to that of Andy Warhol's painting *100 Cans* (1962):

> As dehumanizing and, literally, objectifying as this analogy may seem, the Warhol canvas envisages the form of whatever belonging: difference becomes identical yet remains discreet [*sic*]; units "touch" but do not violate; similitude unbinds the subjects, yet singularity remains intact; relating is not a Venn diagram but bounded. This community, for lack of a better word, has everything and nothing in common; it coheres merely in the form and movement of its seeking. (Roach 2015, 71)

In this way, Grindr users engage in a form of sociality and care that contravenes normative conventions surrounding safe sex negotiation. As discrete entities within a wider social network united by a singular goal, the men's use of words like 'poz' and 'neg' represents an 'attempt to invent a language not yet captured by capital' (Roach 2015, 74). Although this practice might *seem* ruthlessly strategic in nature, it liberates online subjects from potential difficulties surrounding status disclosure, its slangy tone draining safe sex negotiation of its moral weight. Disclosure becomes less about self-management and more about contributing to an esoteric communitarian project in which subjects scatter themselves among scores of online peers in search of mutually satisfactory pleasures.

In facilitating a hookup culture that encourages promiscuity, apps like Grindr transgress neoliberal paradigms reliant on heteronormative coupling and monogamous familial units for their very survival, all while maintaining an alternative language of care to mitigate HIV vulnerabilities within the community. While the neoliberal imperatives that Grindr encourages are incontrovertible, its potential to subvert deeply held tenets of capitalist ideology troubles this reading, revealing a tension I am content to leave unresolved. Indeed, to do otherwise would be to ignore or reduce the often paradoxical nature of the online world (just think, for example, of the broader ways in which online platforms have mobilized counterhegemonic movements like Occupy Wall Street while further entrenching some of neoliberalism's most dehumanizing and immiserating phenomena, such as the deregulation of the labor market through online gig working platforms).

Despite the political complexities surrounding online serosorting as a transmission mitigation method, there is a distinct moralism surrounding online hookup culture that undergirds *Bison*. Take, for example, the following extract which introduces Richard, a gay man in a long-term relationship of over twelve years, who solicits sex from men online:

> [Richard at a mirror. Three males appear but are only partially visible, they are their on-line profile pics; a piece of arse, a hard cock and a shaved off buff chest or something.]
> 1 u online?/
> 4 online u?/
> 2 u online?/
> 1 online u?
> 2 tallhairymuscletop?/
> 1 shavedslutpigbottomboi/
> 1/2 online? (Philpott 2010, 31–2)

Unlike the gestural, carnal sexuality evident in the men awaiting their results, the sexuality of these online users is shaped by the abstractions of digital media. The body becomes purely an end goal to be 'earned' or seduced as its role as mediator is eliminated, thereby facilitating only a one-way form of somatic communication: the body becomes a static signifier of sexual availability and attractiveness. The stage directions embody such dynamics: the fact that the nameless males are partially visible – reduced to what they see as their most alluring, sexual body parts – acts as a kind of visual metaphor for the reductionist, superficial aspects of social media. Furthermore, the fact that, as the playtext states, these men '*are* their on-line profile pics' (Philpott 2010, 31, emphasis my own) reveals the extent to which they see themselves as commercial entities: their online selves are ultimately one and the same as their 'real-world' selves. That Richard is looking at himself in the mirror as he interacts with site users is a particularly telling piece of staging: he lends some attention to his online interlocutors but at the same time is almost entirely focused on himself and the marketability of his own body.

Later in the scene, Richard's essential isolation from the men with whom he interacts becomes clear through some apparently monologic asides related to his boyfriend:

> R Pete and I live together. Have lived together for twelve years. We have a mortgage. Friends of ours put their money up their noses but we…

> 1 Want to fuck or what? Wired with a big pink plank of throbbing meat and a load to shoot right now now now
> R We go shopping every Saturday morning. There's usually cute men… Supermarket's changed hands three times but we have been faithful… well, we've stayed together
> 4 thanks for checking me out you dirty slut dog man woof woof/. (Philpott 2010, 33)

The sexual solicitations of the online platform users with whom he engages are presented more as distractions from his story than as fully realized characters, something reflected by the fact that Richard is afforded a name, while the other men are, again, only numbers. Furthermore, the fact that Richard's replies are utter non sequiturs is evidence of a kind of oblivious egocentricity. In this way, the self-serving individualism of online hookup applications represents a driving force behind the play's politics; a kind of hedonistic and solipsistic subjectivity that the architecture of digital technologies only compounds. It is much easier, after all, to ignore the sexually explicit requests of potential lovers when mediated via the faceless interface of a phone screen.

If there were any doubt as to *Bison*'s ideological bent, Philpott has provided commentary about the beliefs undergirding his play for an academic article, explaining:

> Out of sight out of mind it seems and so everyone goes and fucks bareback and thinks it's okay [...] My feeling is that it is like some huge unspoken suicide mission of the next generation because common sense has been thrown aside for a hedonistic lifestyle and the assumption that PEP [post-exposure prophylaxis] will save them and if that doesn't work it hardly matters anyway because nobody gets ugly lesions and dies from it now anyway. (Campbell 2011, 205–6)

Such sentiments betray a moralism distinctly concomitant of neoliberal health paradigms, demonizing service users who require prescriptions for expensive medicines in order to tackle health issues deemed 'avoidable'. The term 'common sense', while not precisely defined in the context of this extract, seems coterminous with the normative rhetoric of safety problematized by scholars such as Dean and Race. Philpott's invective against contemporary gay culture reveals a neoliberal rationalism that venerates personal responsibility surrounding health and wellbeing while critiquing the objectifying, self-promotional functionality of digital hookup culture. While *Bison* might appear to undermine the self-promotional imperatives undergirding neoliberal appeals to a (phantasmatic) free market, it fails to critique the attendant governance strategies that rigidify neoliberal hegemony. More specifically, it avoids critiquing the delimitation of sexual and somatic freedoms via the promotion of nuclear kinship structures and the demonization of so-called 'lifestyle choices' that supposedly threaten state healthcare provisions.

Of course, there are material and professional benefits associated with staging work that promotes neoliberal health paradigms, demonstrated in part by the corporate funding channeled into Hall's *As Much As I Can*, discussed in the previous chapter. Similarly, theatrical productions treating related themes to *Bison* and *5 Guys Chillin'*, such as Patrick Cash's *The HIV Monologues* (2016) – which critiques digital hookup culture in the context of increasingly strained HIV services – often attract relationships with institutions established to propagate normative public health tenets. Productions of Cash's play, for example, have included post-show Q&As with sexual health experts. The show even headlined the British HIV Association (BHIVA) World AIDS Day Event in 2017, lending institutional backing to a rather simplistic depiction of technology's potential for harm and placing it in tacit agreement with mainstream medical discourses. Indeed, one wonders whether the play's relative critical success (it enjoyed runs at London's Ace Hotel and 503 Theatre, as well as at various queer events and medical conferences) is attributable at least in part to support from medical authorities.

It should come as no surprise, perhaps, that more hegemonically aligned plays are able to gain access to arts institutions and their increasingly paltry funding pots. In commissioning and staging such work, institutions can justify their existence in pragmatic and economic terms, in much the same way that universities and other arts institutions are under pressure to demonstrate the so-called 'impact' of their output through functionalist terms that prioritize metrics like 'value for money'.

Alternative approaches to HIV, health, and community

The impetus behind my critique of public-health-oriented HIV/AIDS plays is by no means to undermine the value of health-related pedagogy in and of itself. Rather, it is to critique how certain plays default to normative scientific and sociopolitical paradigms as a means to mitigate the spread of HIV, such that individualist, alienating, and puritanical forms of queer sociality seem like the only possible common-sense solutions. As with any problem whose causes offend hegemonic interests, remediation necessitates critical approaches to pedagogy and knowledge production that assess how social power dynamics might shape such solutions. As Donna Haraway's well-cited theorization of 'situated knowledges' makes clear, 'admitted or not, politics and ethics ground struggles over knowledge projects in the exact, social, and human sciences' (Haraway 1988, 587), mediated as such projects are by partial perspectives fomented within highly specific sociopolitical worlds. This is not an injunction to relativism, but an alternative approach to knowledge production and discovery that privileges 'partial, locatable, critical knowledges sustaining the possibility of webs of connections called solidarity in politics and shared conversations in epistemology' (Haraway 1988, 584). Such an approach is, of course, incompatible with ways of seeing that privilege personal testimony as incontestable and sacrosanct, as in the aforementioned documentary-style dramaturgies. Indeed, we 'are not immediately present to ourselves. Self-knowledge requires a semiotic-material technology to link meanings and bodies. Self-identity is a bad visual system' (Haraway 1988, 585). While an individual might provide valuable contributions to discourses about public health, their experiences and views are necessarily shaped by wider social forces beyond their control, some of which might contain kernels of prejudice and parochialism. So, how to navigate such tricky epistemic and political terrain while HIV remains a disproportionate worry for variously subjugated sections of society?

In a historical moment saturated by the interests of capital, the possibilities for generative and dialectical approaches to ethical and social problems are necessarily circumscribed. While the stage might *appear* to be a community-oriented space for free thought and countercultural expression, we have already established that the neoliberal dynamics roiling through theaters, their wider institutional networks, and society at large complicate this straightforward assumption. However, this is not to say that the HIV/AIDS genre is devoid of work offering alternative approaches to HIV prevention and knowledge production. One performer who is clearly invested in sparking more generative conversations about HIV with their audiences is David Hoyle, an artist known for his regular performances at both small queer venues and larger, nationally recognized theaters – often as 'anti-drag' queen The Divine David. Hoyle diverges from many of the cultural producers mentioned in this book as he is not, strictly speaking, a playwright. A recent article casts him as an 'underground drag-inflected performer and artist' whose work is largely improvisational and driven by moments of audience interaction (Gallant 2022). As we will see, Hoyle's fringe status and free-wheeling approach to performance have allowed him to critique some of society's more oppressive forms of common sense and, indeed, the very institutions that have facilitated his rise to minor stardom.

Hoyle's *Magazine*, a series of solo performance works that took place at the Royal Vauxhall Tavern between July and September 2007 that each addressed a different (and politically loaded) topic, is exemplary of this kind of resistance from within, with one of its instalments – entitled 'HIV ünt AIDS' – specifically taking aim at neoliberal forms of community-based health messaging about the HIV epidemic. The show itself comprised segments of direct autobiographical address, a video of Hoyle undergoing an HIV test, and an opportunity for individual audience members to take part in onstage conversations with the performer. As demonstrated in footage of the performance, Hoyle starts the show by immediately unsettling and subverting the venue's reputed collective spirit, noting, 'this is a very collective event tonight, ladies and gentleman, the emphasis very much on the "communal" [brief pause]. TOTAL SILENCE now, please. If you wanna have chit chat or talk about what you ate last night for your tea, leave the auditorium immediately' (Jaymes 2007a, 0:14–0:39). Hoyle's instant switch from emphasizing the communal to peremptorily insisting on the full attention of his audience highlights the problematic (perhaps even cynical) use of testimony as representative of a wider community. The jarring interjection of 'TOTAL SILENCE' wittily points out to audience members that Hoyle is ultimately in control of the evening's trajectory, thereby compromising his previous claims to communality and revealing the one-way relationship at their heart.

Building on this premise, Hoyle goes on to interrogate the notion that autobiographical testimony can generate productive alliances between audience members through affective recognition and shared experience. He states:

> This isn't theatre, by the way, ladies and gentleman, this is truth. When you're in a pantomime costume and you're acting and you're doing it all, of course it's beautiful. But occasionally, truth is more important than theatre [pronounced 'tee-a-truh']. And I know that all of us are quite sensitive people who might have been told negative things when they were younger. And that has clouded our vision and made us feel a little bit unworthy and that maybe we should die. (Jaymes 2007b, 0:15–0:54)

While Hoyle's claim to truth might at first appear straightforwardly earnest, his characteristically ironic cadences soon creep in. Hoyle's playful mispronunciation of the word 'theater' indicates that his speech might not be utterly sincere, and his subsequent teasing categorization of every audience member into a group of 'sensitive people' questioning whether they deserve to live affirms such suspicions. While feelings of worthlessness and suicidal thoughts might well reflect Hoyle's own personal past experiences, the notion that all audience members have at some point felt exactly the same way is clearly intended as farce. We might infer at this point a consciousness of the epistemic utility of 'situated knowledges' and, by extension, a critique of the documentary-style queer dramaturgies that, at their worst, might tip into the realms of reactionary moral panic. Hoyle at once pays credence to the very real issues affecting some members of the ill-defined community he addresses, while revealing the folly of leaning on spokespeople to reveal broader so-called 'truths'.

After conveying an obviously sweeping and unqualified assertion, Hoyle uses comedic understatement to signal its absurdity, sardonically linking suicidal ideation to simply feeling 'a little bit unworthy'. In so doing, Hoyle encourages the audience to actively question his role as performer and arbiter of information about HIV/AIDS. Although he ostensibly performs as himself and appears to offer up moments of autobiographical testimony, Hoyle's work is deeply ironical in a way that forces spectators to interrogate the validity of his claims, particularly in regard to notions of blanket identitarian 'truths' and, indeed, heuristic notions of community. In this way, it could be argued that the theatrical project undergirding 'HIV ünt AIDS' and other instalments of Hoyle's *Magazine* is one that attempts to deconstruct from within the auditorium the perceived benefits of testimonial theater that takes on the form of public service announcements, particularly in relation to subcultural performances designed to 'speak back' to the mainstream.

Stephen Greer conceptualizes Hoyle's solo performance project as that of the so-called 'conscious pariah', a figure who challenges claims to collective injury and radicalism that are imbricated within the discourse of marginalized communities, while simultaneously denouncing elements of prevailing hegemonic ideology. Hoyle embodies this figure, Greer argues, thanks to his 'acerbic critique of homogenised desire and homonormative consumerism within mainstream gay culture [that] is inflected by an awareness of the performer's own complicity within those same discourses of desire, and the fragility of his own capacity to enact radical alternatives'

(Greer 2018, 82). This critique of homonormative consumerism is most clearly detectable in Hoyle's frequent references to the £5.99 tickets that audience members were required to purchase in order to gain admission to his performance. At one point during the audience participation segment of the show, Hoyle asks someone he has invited to the stage to talk about their personal experiences regarding safe sex and HIV testing. He asks the participant why they decided to take a test, then quickly turns to the audience to quip 'It's a very psychological study that we're going for for £5.99 tonight' (NewMagazine 2007, 05:32–05:36). In this way, Hoyle expresses a degree of ambivalence about the politics of his work. On the one hand, he seems genuinely interested in nurturing an environment in which HIV testing can be talked about openly in a bid to reduce stigma and suffering, something explicitly asserted at the beginning of the show in the statement: 'I think collectively we can find out procedures for living, for supporting one another, for being' (Jaymes 2007c, 03:51–04:01).

On the other hand, however, Hoyle's show is haunted by its implication within neoliberal structures and, by extension, the ways in which capitalism shapes his relationship with audience members. Lurking beneath his witty references to ticket costs are questions surrounding whether we should put a price on a person's testimony and the ways in which doing so necessarily positions audience members as consumers. Hoyle expresses ambivalence toward these issues by modulating affective community discourse with regular ironic interjections, reminding the audience of the material conditions of his performance and the fact that his decision to perform necessitates that he forsake his widely known political desire to 'ban capitalism – the cruellest, most insulting system any so-called civilisation could choose to impose upon itself' (Hoyle qtd. in Milazzo 2011).

Ultimately, Hoyle's clear discomfort and ambivalence surrounding the theatrical institution within which he is mired seem to be irresolvable. Or rather, he is unable to offer alternative structures. As Daniel Oliver puts it, Hoyle embraces a kind of fragile didacticism that works as 'an affirmation of the ambiguities, fragments and contradictions that arise through the impossibility of any project or cause to be totally stable and uncompromised' (Oliver 2014, 115). Nowhere is this better demonstrated than at the end of 'HIV ünt AIDS': following a bitter diatribe about the ways in which LGBT people celebrate the superficial freedoms that capitalism has granted in order to involve them in consumerism, Hoyle promptly reassures the audience that 'I'll be back. I do believe in value for money' (Jaymes 2007b, 04:52–04:56). While distinguishing himself as a cheap act is, of course, ironic and comically self-deprecating, Hoyle's quick reassurance of repeat performances also indicates that he identifies political, social, and pedagogical value in his work. Although the collective politics 'for living, for supporting one another, for being' might be always fractured by neoliberal imperatives, his self-reflexive recognition of this fact represents a dramaturgy that moves toward communality; that makes the best of the institutional resources available and necessarily consents to certain hegemonic structures to help spark dialectical, movement-building discussion surrounding HIV/AIDS.

In a break from other HIV/AIDS plays examined in this study so far, Hoyle's performances deconstruct the ideological framework shaping even subcultural arts institutions such as the Royal Vauxhall Tavern and, indeed, the 'communities' that form around them. While the notion of a coherent queer community that lies counter to mainstream society might be quixotic or misguided, he suggests, the venue provides fertile ground to isolate and discuss some of the most pressing issues faced by HIV-positive individuals in the venue and beyond. Theaters alone cannot fix the overdetermined and systemic problems that have allowed the HIV epidemic to harm marginalized and subjugated constituencies. However, they might provide the space for mutually constitutive forms of learning and knowledge production. In Haraway's words, they might help us understand '*how* to see from below' and engage in a 'practice of objectivity that privileges contestation, deconstruction, passionate construction, webbed connection, and hopes for transformation of systems of knowledge and ways of seeing' (Haraway 1988, 584–5).

CHAPTER FIVE

Funding HIV/AIDS Theater

Consistent with neoliberalism's addictive imperative to privatize any public good capable of turning a profit, governments across the Global North have spent decades withdrawing increasingly large sums of state funding from the arts and cultural sectors. In the UK, for example, Arts Council England (ACE) – set up in 1946 to support public participation in the arts – has endured a succession of drastic cuts justified by the governmental rhetoric of 'efficiency'. In 2010, for example, the organization's funding was cut by around 30% (Higgins 2010), while more recent government reviews have raised the prospect of abolishing ACE altogether (Harris 2022). At the same time, access to other forms of state support for those out of work has been eroded, often replaced by punitive welfare legislation demanding constant subjugation to bureaucratic employment agencies. As a result, securing the resources and institutional backing necessary to stage new plays has become an increasingly challenging, competitive, and thankless affair for those without access to private wealth, elite professional networks, and the means to reproduce oneself without engaging in time-consuming wage labor.

As the late Mark Fisher lamented, neoliberalism has deprived artists of the material resources necessary for generating and engaging with new cultural forms (Fisher 2014, 24). While marketized, profit-driven sectors are incentivized to churn out films, TV shows, and albums resembling successfully tried-and-tested cultural products, creative types are increasingly unable to risk withdrawing from the traditional labor market to cultivate their skills – damaging the pipeline that might eventually funnel amateur and independent artists into more mainstream and widely celebrated cultural realms. Indeed,

> It's no accident that the efflorescence of cultural invention in London and New York in the late 1970s and early 80s (in the punk and postpunk scenes) coincided with the availability of squatted and cheap property in those cities. Since then, the decline of social housing, the attacks on squatting, and the delirious rise in property prices have meant that the amount of time and energy available for cultural production has massively diminished. (Fisher 2014, 24)

Such a combination of morbid symptoms raises questions about the trajectory of HIV/AIDS theater in recent decades. With fewer traditional funding pots available to create art and theater, many playwrights have turned to alternative models such as crowdfunding to support their work.

In this chapter, I will examine the consequences of these shifts for HIV/AIDS theater (and, by implication, the theater landscape more broadly). As revivals of major hits such as *Angels in America* subsume the vast majority of funding propping up HIV/AIDS theater, how do newer playwrights position themselves and their work in relation to the art of the so-called 'crisis years'? Furthermore, given the existence of protease inhibitors in the twenty-first century, how do these playwrights justify the funding of their work in a neoliberal culture obsessed with metrics, productivity, and 'usefulness'? And, finally, to what extent is there scope for artistic dissidence in a socio-economic environment so adept at draining its working classes of time, money, energy, and willingness to fight their own exploitation? In answering these questions, we might disinter how neoliberalism's material rapaciousness has affected the themes and political messaging detectable in contemporary HIV/AIDS plays, as well as the accessibility of these plays for mainstream audiences.

Promises, pledges, and shoestring budgets: crowdfunding HIV/AIDS theater in a post-crash economy

Many of the first HIV/AIDS playwrights faced a rather different funding environment to today's generation. *Angels in America*, for example, reached the cultural stature it enjoys today as a result of funding from the National Endowment for the Arts (NEA) in the US. As Tony Kushner noted in a recent published oral history of the play, 'the NEA offered this $50,000 dollar grant, and $40,000 would go to production. That was more money than I'd ever made for anything

[...] I was sort of being commissioned to write – the federal government's commissioning me to write – a play.' (qtd. in Butler and Kois 2018, 34–5). To put this into context, the grants originally promised to the NEA Four amounted to between $5,000 and $11,250 each (Span and Hall 1990) – smaller figures that better reflect what artists could expect to receive at the time. Even today, average NEA grants amount to only $23,190 for organizations or established projects (National Endowment for the Arts 2021). So, while Kushner's grant might not have delivered instant riches, its relative generosity represented a willingness to take risks on new and upcoming artists that has all but disappeared in today's hostile funding environment.

Much like ACE, money has gradually been sucked from the NEA over the past few decades, in no small part due to the economic turmoil precipitated by the global financial crisis of 2008. According to a report by Americans for the Arts, the NEA would have received $320.7 million in 2019 if funding had remained constant since 1992 (adjusting for inflation). In actuality, it received only $155 million (Cohen 2019). The paltriness of this funding pot can also be traced back beyond the financial crash to the infamous NEA Four row, which emerged out of America's culture wars in the 1990s and resulted in funding being withdrawn from individual artists (as explored in Chapter 2). Inevitably, one wonders whether a young Kushner would have gained access to such a healthy grant in today's world, scarred as it is by deep cuts to the arts and other social goods. While we cannot answer this question with any certainty, it seems highly unlikely that he and other accomplished playwrights of his generation would have had such easy access to federal funds in less favorable economic circumstances. By extension, we might doubt whether Kushner would have been able to write such a wildly popular and thematically rich play as *Angels* if confronted with the challenges today's playwrights face.

Of course, we must not lose sight of the political limitations of state support for cultural production. State grants are not 'gifts', tied as they are to both official and tacit productivity (or 'impact') requirements. For example, while *Angels* presents a critical, even caustic, image of Reaganite America in the 1980s, controversies surrounding artists the NEA chose to fund in the 1990s suggest that Kushner's work would not have enjoyed such generous funding if it had transgressed certain normative boundaries. Certainly, the calls for progress, tolerance, and even gradualism in *Angels* appear to contain a type of pluralism far more consistent with hegemonic ideologies than, say, the resolutely queer, utopian politics seen in works like Tim Miller's *My Queer Body* (examined in Chapter 2). Miller received NEA funding that was later rescinded due to the protestatory nature of his work, effectively publicizing the federal establishment's contempt for AIDS activists. To some extent, the controversy surrounding Miller's work served his communitarian form of performance well, compelling him to seek out cheap – and thereby intimate – venues in which bonds between audience members could be nurtured. Furthermore, the unavoidably pared-back nature of his productions (props were scant and his body alone became the focal point of the work) lent poignancy to his testimonial monologues and served as a visual metaphor for the government's lack of support for his cause, thereby emphasizing the urgent need for political action to address the crisis.

Other notable examples of HIV/AIDS performers and playwrights whose work was defunded for reasons of 'obscenity' include Karen Finley – whose grant was rescinded for *We Keep Our Victims Ready* (1990), a show about sexual violence and subjugation of (especially racialized) women – and Ron Athey, whose S&M-influenced performance practices included bloodletting, body modification, saline injections, and other pain-inducing activities. While Finley's deeply personal AIDS-related performance pieces, such as *A Certain Level of Denial* (1992), generated intimate spaces to grieve and reflect through stories about the untimely deaths of many of her friends, Athey's work was more confrontational and focused on engaging its audience in sensual and transgressive experiences. HIV-positive himself, Athey's performances highlighted the pain inflicted on people with AIDS by neglectful governments while defending their autonomy as erotic and sexual beings. Jesse Helms described Athey as a 'human cockroach' in response to such explicit work (Shanks 2018), which was often shot through with religious iconography, casting the artist as a depraved harbinger of the downfall of American civilization. Capitalizing on the controversy, Helms used Athey's demonization as fuel in his campaign to defund the NEA, consistently reminding the American public that their tax dollars went toward supporting Athey's work.

As Dominic Johnson notes, citing Jonathan Dollimore, figures like Helms fought so vociferously for a notion of art as a respectable vehicle for esthetic pleasure and social cohesion – rather than a challenging political force – because the incitement of emotions such as disgust and anger could effectively garner opposition to hegemonic norms. Indeed, the 'oppositional potential of Athey's work was registered most keenly by government officials, and policed as though it signified the violent force of a return of the repressed' (Johnson 2013, 86). While the work of Miller, Finley, and Athey differs significantly in content and style, its ability to instill fear in government officials lays bare some of the challenges artists faced in gathering the resources necessary to stage oppositional work that was willing to test and confront audiences. More than a fact of simple economics, public funding for HIV/AIDS theater was saturated with political weight and served as a measure of the extent to which playwrights and their plays were ideologically compatible with contemporary neoliberalism.

For all the ingenuity and resourcefulness evident in the work of oppositional and defunded performers, however, we must avoid romanticizing the plight of the struggling artist. While shoestring budgets might compel theater makers to experiment with dramaturgical techniques, the ability of these artists to reach large audiences is severely curtailed compared to their generously funded counterparts. In any political project oriented toward coalition building and consciousness raising, the ability to reach wide audiences represents a fundamental element of success. Returning again to the case of *Angels*, for example, federal funding allowed Kushner's play to grace the Broadway stage and eventually be adapted for TV audiences in 2003 – allowing, as one *Los Angeles Times* journalist put it, the play's 'intertwined metaphors' to 'inhabit America's dens and bedrooms' (Stayton 2003). In a bid to maximize exposure and ignite public conversations, therefore, many of today's political theater makers are turning to alternative sources to fund and popularize their plays.

Somewhat inevitably, the emergence of the internet as by far the most powerful resource for disseminating information and organizing social projects in the late twentieth and early twenty-first centuries presented new opportunities for cash-strapped artists. While academics and thinkers of all political shades have thrown the supposed liberatory potential of digital media into serious doubt over the past couple of decades, the internet's capabilities for data exchange are undeniable.[1] On a broad level, this function has spawned new economic possibilities in the Global North, including the inception of the online sharing, platform, and gift economies. The scope of the so-called sharing economy is very broad, and basically encompasses any online activity involving an exchange of commodities that falls outside traditional business models (i.e., an arrangement in which companies hire employees to create and distribute goods and

1 See Nick Srnicek, *Platform Capitalism* (2016); Shoshana Zuboff, *The Age of Surveillance Capitalism* (2018); Richard Seymour, *The Twittering Machine* (2019); Jeremy Gilbert and Alex Williams, *Hegemony Now* (2022) for a taste of recent critiques.

services for consumers). By far the most popular examples of sharing economy platforms are the ride-hailing service Uber and the subletting service Airbnb, both of which connect service users with local service providers operating as self-employed workers. Of course, while these services appear to eliminate the proverbial middleman associated with traditional forms of purchasing, the 'sharing' aspect of this arrangement represents a wild misnomer. As Doug Henwood puts it, 'The sharing economy is a nice way for rapacious capitalists to monetize the desperation of people in the post-crisis economy while sounding generous, and to evoke a fantasy of community in an atomized population' (Henwood, 2015). By turning service providers into mini-entrepreneurs, sharing platforms incentivize workers to adopt increasingly precarious forms of work and relinquish labor rights, while liberating companies who run sharing platforms from various forms of corporate accountability.

The social dynamics of the gift economy, meanwhile, are a little trickier to pin down. While it operates as a subcategory of the sharing economy, gift economy exchanges do not explicitly operate on a (purportedly) *quid pro quo* basis in the same way as services like Uber and Airbnb. Examples of gift economics include the development of open-source software, open-access publishing, peer-to-peer lending platforms, or crowdfunding websites. On the one hand, open-source sites such as Wikipedia – an online encyclopedia reliant on user contributions – appear to democratize access to knowledge and other digital assets. On the other hand, as we will soon explore, the notion of the 'gift economy' is bound up with complex social dynamics that, as with the term 'sharing economy', bely its stated function. What appears free at face value might come with alternative obligations and compromises that serve the interests of capital despite a lack of direct monetary exchange.

From the viewpoint of the 2020s, big tech platforms and their atomizing imperatives have clearly had a profound impact on capitalism's contemporary dynamics. For some, tech companies' ability to catalyze exploitation rates might indicate their capture of a new phase of capitalist hegemony (Gilbert and Williams 2022, 199). It is unsurprising, therefore, that the theater industry has been altered by certain aspects of the new digital economy. One of the most significant shifts related to the funding and staging of new plays is the emergence of crowdfunding platforms. Put simply, crowdfunding involves the online collection of donations to fund a project or venture, and has markedly impacted how some theater productions, particularly those on the fringes of the mainstream, are funded and produced in the twenty-first century. As we will see, crowdfunding is imbued with capitalist logic – a kind of patch or salve to cover up some of the deepest wounds that neoliberalism has inflicted on the cultural sphere. What makes the phenomenon so worthy of examination in the context of HIV/AIDS theater is the fact that so many playwrights in the genre are (however deliberately) committed to tackling the problems driven or exacerbated by contemporary capitalism. Are there contradictions between crowdfunding and staging counterhegemonic plays? Does crowdfunding encourage certain forms of assimilationist art? And does the rise of crowdfunding risk further decimating available arts funding by legitimizing autonomous fundraising as quick, effective, and unbound from state interests?

Within the realm of HIV/AIDS theater, several playwrights have managed to secure a platform and an audience for their works thanks to the donations of crowdfunders. Examples include Neil Watkins' *The Year of Magical Wanking* (2010), the GHP Collective's *The Gay Heritage Project* (2013), Nathaniel Hall's *First Time* (2018), and Shaun Kitchener's *Positive* (2015), a British production that first gained exposure at the Edinburgh Fringe Festival and will provide a focus for the first half of this chapter. Given this production's location, the discussion that follows will center primarily on the UK economy and funding structures. However, while there are, of course, variations in the proportion of public to private funding between different countries (the NEA in the US, for example, is known for being particularly parsimonious compared to its European equivalents), I view the motivating factors driving the rise of crowdfunding as transnational phenomena. Generally speaking, playwrights and performance artists across the Global North have had to negotiate a leaner public funding environment since the dawn of the new millennium compared to that of the latter decades of the twentieth century, something digital pioneers have been addressing (indeed, exploiting) through the creation of crowdfunding platforms. At the same time, however, the ever-tightening grip of neoliberal ideology is driving the rise of what could be termed the 'consumer-philanthropist', a person who donates to artistic endeavors seemingly out of pure generosity while expecting a particular reward or gift in return.

To disentangle the social relations at play in crowdfunding, I turn briefly to Kickstarter – one of the most widely used crowdfunding platforms on the market. Between Kickstarter's founding in April 2009 and April 2023, a total of $44.54 million has been channeled into its 12,959 theater projects worldwide, indicating a high level of motivation among users to help bring underfunded projects to the stage (Kickstarter 2023). Site visitors are given the option to pledge sums of money to a creative project in return for (largely symbolic) rewards. Those who donated £10 or more to *Positive*, for example, were offered recognition on social media, progress rehearsal updates and a copy of the script; those who donated £20 or more were offered all of these rewards as well as a ticket to the performance of their choice; and donors who pledged over £50 were offered two complementary tickets for a performance of their choice, a signed copy of the script, and a personalized recorded song of thanks.

Of course, one of the main questions to emerge out of the crowdfunding phenomenon is why participants choose to donate money, however small the sum, in return for rewards that have a much lower market value (if any). Excluding donors who face social pressures seemingly extraneous to market logic such as obligations to friends and family, crowdfunders appear to subvert the core neoliberal tenet of profitability and self-interest, indicating that their motivations might lie within prosocial rather than individualistic realms. In the context of HIV/AIDS theater, then, donating could indicate a desire to help theater makers disseminate information about HIV/AIDS and reduce associated stigma among a theatergoing public, something that has, to varying degrees, been a central element of the genre since its inception. The rubric of Kitchener's Kickstarter page for *Positive*, for example, certainly appears to cater to this kind of sentiment:

> HIV is a thing. It's a thing that isn't necessarily as scary a thing as it once was but it's certainly a bigger thing than you may well think it is. You with me?
>
> *Positive* is a play about Benji. He's in his mid-twenties, and he's an ordinary chap trying to make his way through life, love and all that malarkey in modern-day Britain. He is also one of 100,000 people living in this country right now with HIV (or at least he would be if he wasn't fictional). (Kitchener n.d.)

Kitchener's conversational tone and gentle probing of his readers ('You with me?') seemingly demonstrates an attempt to build a collaborative relationship with funders. At its starkest level, such a rubric is designed to appeal to the charitable, prosocial sensibilities of crowdfunding website users interested in contributing to a project that raises awareness of the contemporary realities of HIV, particularly those for whom the statistics provided might come as a shock.

Perhaps unsurprisingly, however, raising a critical anti-capitalist lens to the fundraising page for *Positive* rather complicates this one-dimensional reading of crowdfunders' motivations. If we adhere to a simplistic and fundamentalist conception of the neoliberal world, the practice of contributing to a crowdfund appears illogical, as individuals are essentially entrepreneurial entities by default. As such, we must infer that crowdfunding is either utterly extraneous to the flows of capital (surely difficult, if not impossible, in our networked world) or is undergirded by a deeper nexus of reciprocities and motivations. The inchoate body of scholarly work on crowdfunding and the sharing economy – typically emerging from the fields of sociology or the digital humanities, and highly influenced by the work of French sociologist Marcel Mauss – certainly seems to support the idea that lines between generosity and self-interest become blurred on sites like Kickstarter.[2] Mauss's most famous work, *The Gift* (1925), represents a strong theoretical framework through which to analyze the motivations of the crowdfunder in its stipulation that all gifts are loaded with obligations, social bonds, and reciprocities. The gift is the 'present generously given even when, in the gesture accompanying the transaction, there is only a polite fiction, formalism, and social deceit, and when really there is obligation and economic self-interest' (Mauss [1925] 1990, 4). As such, no gift is truly 'free', and crowdfunding is beleaguered by self-interest on both sides of the equation.

Although Mauss's theories were promulgated in the early twentieth century, long before the inception of Web 2.0, they have only been further corroborated by the public forum of the internet. As Mary Douglas explains in the foreword to a 1990 edition of *The Gift*, Maussian theory stipulates that the

> gift cycle echoes Adam Smith's invisible hand: gift complements market in so far as it operates where the latter is absent. Like the market it supplies each individual with personal incentives for collaborating in the pattern of exchanges. Gifts are given in the context of public drama, with nothing secret about them. In being more directly cued to public esteem, the distribution of honour, and the sanctions of religion, the gift economy is more visible than the market. (Douglas qtd. in Mauss [1925] 1990, xviii)

2 See, for example, André et al.'s 'Beyond the Opposition Between Altruism and Self-interest: Reciprocal Giving in Reward-Based Crowdfunding' (2017)

The internet, then, as a public forum accessible from almost anywhere in the world at any time, heightens this sense of 'public esteem' when it comes to crowdfunding. As demonstrated by Kitchener's entreaty, rewards come not in the form of material gain (only scripts and tickets are offered), but in the form of clout, approbation, and personal promotion (i.e., social media mentions). If self-branding and promotion are central to the cultivation of an entrepreneurial, neoliberal self, then ostensibly altruistic contributions to crowdfunded projects can be problematized by the specter of self-interest.

Furthermore, the spatio-temporal architecture of the contemporary internet is such that the 'public drama' of gift giving has a certain kind of permanence; it is recorded and can be accessed again and again, meaning crowdfunders' public esteem can be reaffirmed inexhaustibly. In this way, while altruism might play at least some part in their reasons for donating to theater projects online, the neoliberal environment that crowdfunders navigate ineluctably shackles their motives to the lure of public recognition. Certainly, the notion that crowdfunders are largely driven by public acknowledgement and esteem is backed up by the prevailing market research surrounding theater funding. In a study of 875 Kickstarter-funded theater projects established between 2011 and 2014, researchers found that the 'propensity to donate is greater when the entrepreneur offers public acknowledgement without material rewards; it is weakest when no rewards are offered at all' (Boeuf et al. 2014, 42). Furthermore, 'material rewards have a negative influence on the number of crowdfunders who choose to support a project in cases where public acknowledgement is offered' (Boeuf et al. 2014, 42). Although the authors of this research posited their findings as evidence of prosocial behavior, the fact that material rewards have a *negative* impact on funding surely demonstrates that many crowdfunders harbor concerns about the potentially reputation-damaging effect of accepting such rewards. Indeed, material rewards might not carry the positive symbolic weight with which they are usually associated in this context, perhaps harboring the ominous potential to mar a person's philanthropic image or 'brand'.

In today's cultural economy, of course, convincing crowdfunders to attach their name to a project about HIV/AIDS might prove tricky. Firstly, there remains a pervasive stigma surrounding HIV, potentially discouraging funders from getting involved. Secondly, the fatal urgency that once surrounded the pandemic and encouraged governmental organizations to fund HIV/AIDS theater has lessened in recent decades, leaving crowdfunders to wonder whether their money would be better utilized on other projects. To maximize their chances of success in a landscape saturated with worthy projects, many of the project starters on crowdfunding sites carefully craft online personas into which funders can 'invest'. Kitchener, for example, preempts some of the reasons funders might not wish to support an HIV/AIDS play and uses this to his advantage in the rubric for *Positive*, which he describes as

> A warm-hearted comedy inspired by true stories, *Positive* is not a dark and gloomy drama about death and disease [...] It's just an entertaining show with a few laughs, a few serious bits and the occasional reference to Britney Spears; designed to shatter the inaccurate preconceptions that A) HIV doesn't really exist in Britain anymore, and B) those who are HIV+ are somehow vastly different to those who aren't. (Kitchener n.d.)

In trivializing the seriousness or importance of his work and distancing himself from the various death-filled plays of the past (an option, perhaps, available only to playwrights of the 'post-crisis' era), Kitchener attends instead to cultivating a likeable, charming online voice, selling his personality as a brand of sorts.

While the pedagogical purpose of *Positive* is clearly imbued with some prosocial intentions, the lack of urgency displayed in Kitchener's rubric along with an 'all or nothing' funding model used by Kickstarter is evidence of an ideological gulf between older and younger generations of HIV/AIDS theater makers. Indeed, Kickstarter does not give any funds to a given project if it does not reach its target goal, a quasi-competitive model that goes against the imperative 'make do' attitude adopted by many second-generation theater makers motivated by the (largely accurate) belief that improving the lives of HIV-positive people would require fighting dominant powers, rather than working within prevailing hegemonic structures.

This gulf is detectable even in recent crowdfunding pitches that adopt a more earnest and urgent approach to the HIV crisis. Nathaniel Hall's crowdfunding page for *First Time*, a solo play about the experience of being diagnosed as a teenager, impresses the importance of the play on crowdfunders by noting:

> we know there are thousands of people across the country who still live in fear of people finding our [*sic*] their HIV status.
>
> Stigmatising headlines are not uncommon, and they add fuel to the fire that people with HIV are a danger to others and contribute to a culture of fear that stops people from getting tested regularly. (Hall 2019)

Much like the public-health-oriented plays I discussed in the preceding chapter, Hall does not address the material bases upon which stigma thrives and, by extension, the ways in which racialized and otherwise marginalized constituencies are rendered more vulnerable to infection. This is not to say that Hall's aims to educate audiences about living with HIV are futile or prejudiced. As a *Gay Times* reviewer noted, the play is 'full of humour, charm and a genuine, honest warmth, as Nathaniel is just such a likeable performer' (Selman 2022) – valuable traits, surely, for the effective dissemination of information about living with HIV in contemporary Britain. However, undergirding Hall's crowdfunding project are loftier aims than changing a few spectators' minds. As the funding page asserts, thanks to 'the introduction of PrEP, more people on effective treatment and better HIV health campaigns, leading charities believe that we now have the tools to end HIV in a generation', with stigma the primary barrier we need to bulldoze to make such an achievement a reality (Hall 2019). In staging *First Time*, Hall and the producers 'want to educate, destigmatise and empower, in turn contributing the aim of ending HIV in a generation [*sic*]' (Hall 2019). In this way, they harness hegemonic public health paradigms surrounding individual responsibility as a means to attract crowdfunders, promoting the show as a potential solution to high transmission rates.

As the preceding chapters in this book have hopefully clarified, the continued proliferation of HIV and the disproportionate ways in which it affects the world's subaltern majority are necessarily enmeshed within capitalist logics. While we might indeed have the *tools* to quell transmission rates, we currently lack the distributive societal structures necessary to maximize their efficacy and to care for those most vulnerable to HIV/AIDS – a fact that crowdfunded plays obscure through normative teleologies of progress and undeniably neoliberal forms of individualism. While contemporary HIV/AIDS playwrights are afforded a wider variety of funding options in our digitally networked century, the technologies that facilitate such opportunities are imbued with social relations that shape the conception and content of the plays themselves. For example, while we cannot claim that *Positive* was written and produced solely in line with the needs of consumer-philanthropists, the play's optimistic branding and light, inoffensively humorous content undeniably sit well within a crowdfunding model. After all, as Kitchener himself notes on his Kickstarter page, '[a]side from the budget, an obvious concern with taking a show to the Fringe is actually getting an audience in to see the damn thing' (Kitchener n.d.). This throws up a number of questions about the rising number of crowdfunded HIV/AIDS plays. Are funding models to some extent 'mainstreaming' the content of new plays? And is the competitive element of sites like Kickstarter creating a novel funding model that is increasingly hewn out of a brutely commercial mold?

Perhaps unsurprisingly, given the seductive, seemingly emancipatory potentialities that inhere within the online world, several academics and theater critics would answer such questions emphatically in the negative, instead championing Kickstarter as a galvanizing counterhegemonic force. Paul Langley and Andrew Leyshon, for example, believe that

> crowdfunding appears as something of an antidote to the oligopolistic concentration and centralization of capital investment, a digital economy that necessarily cuts against the grain of the mainstream and the traditional, and which has the remedial and ameliorative capacity to make funding available to individuals and institutions that would otherwise be excluded from capital allocations. (Langley and Leyshon 2017, 1023)

This view is supported by the increasing number of theater makers able to fully realize their projects by way of crowdfunding. As early as 2012, Kickstarter was already on its way to channeling more money into arts projects than the NEA in the US (Rosen 2012), an upward trend reflected globally that has benefited amateur playwrights such as Kitchener.

However, such a thesis is fraught with problems, given crowdfunding's ineluctable ties to self-interest and promotion. While crowdfunding has delivered novel opportunities for people outside of the professional art world to choose which plays get funded, it has done so in an atomized fashion that ignores social responsibilities and interrelatedness. Funders need not interact or work together to discuss the merits of funding a particular play, 'despite the intimation of co-activity and potential collectivism in the word "crowd". Crowdfunding also risks, again, legitimating the rolling back of state support for the arts by stepping in to fill its gaps' (Harvie 2013, 173). As such, the paradoxically isolating yet socially inclusive spatio-temporality of online space amplifies neoliberalism's individualizing tenets. Rather than the 'crowd' operating as a cohesive community supportive of general principles, it is structured as a collection of distinct actors focused on their individual needs and desires. A funding model drained of 'mutual social responsibility' emulates the architecture of the neoliberal free market, leaving theater makers with an abundance of factors to consider if they want to be successful in their funding efforts. For a genre such as HIV/AIDS theater, this trend is particularly stifling, as playwrights appear compelled to promote their embryonic projects through the rubric of public health and pedagogy, something that goes a long way to explaining why the counterhegemonic fervor of second-generational plays faded away at the dawn of the millennium. If, as Jen Harvie suggests, crowdfunding legitimizes the decimation of public arts funding, its persistent rise is surely poised to encourage the creation of increasingly 'safe' and commercialized HIV/AIDS theater that avoids the risk of critical rejection.

The significant influence on crowdfunding on the shape of HIV/AIDS theater does not preclude the conditions for counterhegemonic work, of course. Perhaps the best means for penny-pinching artists to launch their work onto the stage is through solo performance. Often deemed a germane genre for giving counterhegemonic forms of testimony a platform, solo performance complicates the reading of contemporary HIV/AIDS plays as immanently more susceptible to hegemonic influences than their predecessors. As such, I turn my attention to Neil Watkins' crowdfunded play, *The Year of Magical Wanking*, to examine the extent to which solo practitioners are motivated and, indeed, able to subvert the constrictions of the neoliberal theater sector.

'I wank, therefore I slam': Neil Watkins' *The Year of Magical Wanking*

The solo performance has long been a mainstay of political queer theater. On one level, we can view the trend for solo work as grounded in brute economics. Lacking the funds necessary to stage large productions, impecunious artists might turn to the solo form for politically urgent ends; to spread a clear message quickly without having to wait for institutional or monetary support. However, as Deirdre Heddon explains, the links between autobiographical solo performance and queerness are also traceable to a desire to resist marginalization and claim agency within a heteronormative and heterosexist society. 'Autobiographical performances', she writes, 'provide a way to talk out, talk back, talk otherwise. Here, the marginalised subject can literally take centre stage' (Heddon 2008, 3). Similarly, in the dialogic introduction to Holly Hughes and David Román's anthology of queer monologic works, *O Solo Homo: The New Queer Performance* (1998), the pair discuss how solo performance is historically entwined with the country's social change movements, as exemplified in Hughes's own autobiographical work *Clit Notes* (1996), in which she wryly speaks out against her own marginalization at the hands of both homophobic family members and national institutions such as the NEA. Expanding on this point in a conversation with Hughes, Román states that the trend is indicative of a distinctly queer desire for identity and community. He argues that 'queer solo performers trouble the comfort of community even as they invest in it [...] One could even argue that queer solo performers are often at the frontiers of new social identities and more inclusive community formations' (Hughes and Román 1998, 5–6).

Tying such assertions together is a faith in the galvanizing role of 'community' in solo performance – specifically, queer community. Although the term is fairly polysemic, the scholars clearly gesture toward community's reparative conceptualization as a space for similarly identified or politically affiliated individuals to resist their oppression by the forces of prevailing hegemony. Heddon's claim that autobiographical performance offers historically marginalized artists the opportunity to 'talk out' and 'talk back' gestures toward a quasi-reciprocal (rather than merely presentational) performer–spectator relationship. She goes on to assert that 'to be part of an audience is potentially to be allied with others', a communal relationship reinforced by solo performance's often conversational mode of address, as well as a call to establish political affiliations grounded in common experiences of oppression (Heddon 2008, 6). Solo theater's potential to inspire dialogue might indicate why the form has proved so popular among performers affiliated with marginalized identity groups: it feeds into motivations to initiate conversation and action surrounding injustices.

Such a desire is particularly acute for groups affected by HIV/AIDS. As Monica Pearl notes in *AIDS Literature and Gay Identity: The Literature of Loss* (2013), a common trait in the art and literature of the AIDS crisis is a preoccupation with conversation and its potential to structure so-called 'queer filiations' or 'network[s] of friends and chosen families' or, indeed, what we might term 'communities' (Pearl 2013, 150). Citing examples as wide-ranging as the ACT UP Oral History Project, Kushner's *Angels in America*, Eve Kosofsky Sedgwick's *A Dialogue on Love* (1999) and performance installations by the likes of Ron Athey and Lois Weaver, Pearl identifies these works as presenting 'disordered and continuous exchanges and dialogues [that] consolidate community through sustaining loss' (Pearl 2013, 160). In other words, the myriad losses that have been incurred by queer individuals since the emergence of the HIV/AIDS epidemic – such as the loss of friends or lovers, the loss of somatic agency, or the loss of familial ties as a result of phobic rejection – might serve as generative sites of queer kinship and, by extension, political power. Indeed, Pearl identifies the loss of acceptance within normative society as a particularly community-building force, noting that 'outcasts can aspire to be included and recognized by claiming insider or normative status, or else not by repudiating the status of outcast but claiming *community* outcast status' (Pearl 2013, 163).

It should come as no surprise, therefore, that a striking proportion of HIV/AIDS plays and performances have been monologic or solo pieces designed for a single actor, often in relatively intimate settings. Many have been autobiographical or testimonial in nature, such as Miller's *My Queer Body.* Others have been verbatim or testimonial accounts performed by single actors, such as Alexis Gregory's *Riot Act* (2018), which uses interviews from activists and artists (including an AIDS activist) to produce a whistlestop tour of queer history. A consistent theme throughout such testimonial plays is a call – either implicit or explicit – to intracommunity solidarity. As explored in Chapter 2, *My Queer Body* made the most of intimate, low-cost venues to galvanize political fervor and provide members of the queer community (mostly gay men) with opportunities to bond, grieve, and organize. As a twenty-first-century play, Gregory's is markedly different in form and tone, attempting to historicize the 'crisis years' and educate modern audiences about pivotal moments in the history of queer liberation. He performs (or 'channels') the testimony of a Stonewall survivor, an AIDS activist, and a drag artist who launched a career in the squats of 1970s London.

A pedagogical work, Gregory's play can be seen to extend beyond the interests of identitarian community – the limitations of which I discuss at length in Chapter 2 – and encourage audiences to empathize with its subjects as a means to inform their own politics and activism. In an interview, Gregory notes that this pedagogical function was bolstered throughout the tour by workshops 'for LGBTQ+ communities, and our allies, in the areas we visit. The workshops are either writing or performance based, so we'll be […] exploring queer storytelling and representation' (chloethefry 2022). Within the confines of a hegemonic liberal logic, such educational programs work toward liberating the LGBTQ+ from intolerant attitudes and stigmatization within the wider community. As reviewers have noted, *Riot Act* 'powerfully conveyed the pain and trauma of AIDS' (Findlay 2022) and offered 'thoroughly human insights into big moments in queer history;

Stonewall, Liberation, and AIDS' (Garside 2022). Activist Jason Jones noted that 'For me as an activist, this piece represents what all activists ultimately desire, to be heard! These voices need to be heard!' (Jones 2018). Clearly, Gregory's talent as a performer and writer help generate affecting theater that both educates its audience and galvanizes empathy between generations or marginalized constituencies – arguably a vital foundational component in any liberatory project.

However, despite its activist themes and commitment to amplifying historically marginalized voices, Gregory's project is constrained by some of the hegemonic narratives that make queer organizing – and organizing more generally – so difficult in neoliberal times. As well as reifying queer history as coherently teleological and intelligible (rather than unwieldy and contestable) in a similar way to Kramer's *The Normal Heart*, Gregory's impulse to draw distinct lines between LGBTQ+ communities and their 'allies' precludes the development of an anti-capitalist consciousness – which, I have argued, necessitates conceptualizing the relationship between queerness and the normative as always dialectical, dynamic, and unstable.

Although such a distinction might seem insignificant or merely semantic, the notion of allyship often struggles to look beyond neoliberal paradigms of selfhood and sociality. As Jodi Dean explains in her polemical *Comrade* (2019), people who adopt the role of the ally tend to be those with relative economic and social privilege who want to help tackle oppression, regardless of whether they have encountered such oppression themselves. In other words, 'allies can be straight people who stand up for LGBTQ people, white people who support black and brown people, men who defend women, and so on' (Dean 2019, 16). As part of this supportive work, allies are required to listen to – and absorb lessons from – the oppressed, acknowledging their own privilege while allowing others to guide political movements to avoid perpetuating the discriminatory misdeeds of their privileged peers. Under this logic, 'it's as if struggles were possessions – artifacts that individuals take on, over, and into themselves – all while being urged to see these acquisitions as something to which they, as the ally, have no right' (Dean 2019, 18). As such, political consciousness remains within the realm of the imaginary and affective, rather than the material and solidaristic – both vital aspects of counterhegemonic struggle.

While solo testimonial performances like *Riot Act* might help to teach allies a certain version of queer history, therefore, they understandably struggle to identify how the interests of a broad range of constituencies might intersect. One questions, therefore, the extent to which a less didactic and more exploratory, extroverted, risky form of solo HIV theater might generate the kind of anti-capitalist consciousness necessary to appreciate both the pandemic's driving forces and how addressing the ongoing crisis requires deep, transformational change in how society is run – change that, ultimately, will serve all but its upper echelons. As Dean explains, 'If we recognize that the attachment to individual identity is the form of our political incapacity, we can acquire new capacities for action, the collective capacities of those on the same side of a struggle' (Dean 2019, 22).

While my review of solo HIV/AIDS theater is unavoidably and necessarily partial (texts, recordings, and reviews of shoestring plays are notoriously difficult to unearth), I have identified at least one play that avoids interpellating audiences as members or allies of bounded community – Neil Watkins' *The Year of Magical Wanking* (2011). Another crowdfunded play, *TYoMW* uses the solo form to universalize certain forms of struggle and raise consciousness of neoliberalism's alienating imperatives. It was produced on a slim budget of €6,000 and rejects the pedagogical imperatives of plays like *Positive*. First performed at Ireland's Queer Notions festival in 2010, *TYoMW* can best be described as a (mostly) autobiographical poetic monologue exploring a year in Watkins' life as a 33-year-old, HIV-positive gay man living in Dublin. It tracks the twelve months following Watkins' diagnosis as he spends a considerable amount of time depressed and alone in his deceased grandfather's flat, failing to connect with old friends or new lovers and struggling with drug addiction. That Watkins is the same age as Jesus when he died is no coincidence here, as he figures himself as a kind of prophetic martyr sent to warn others against making the same life-altering mistakes as his younger self, blaming such mistakes, in part, on feelings of personal shame instilled by a strict Catholic upbringing.

The play is deeply intertextual, referring not only to Catholic tradition but to myriad religious, spiritual, and cultural phenomena both mainstream and obscure. One example of such intertextuality is the work's title, which is, of course, a play on Joan Didion's *The Year of Magical Thinking* (2005), an autobiographical performance describing the author's experiences of grief surrounding the death of her husband in 2003 and scrutinizing her own emotional instability in the year leading up to the event. Before the play even begins, therefore, this literary allusion prepares the audience for themes surrounding mourning and loss. That Watkins replaces the word 'thinking' with the less delicate 'wanking', however, also alerts us to its comic overtones and potential for bathos. On the one hand, *TYoMW* could be compared to Tim Miller's *My Queer Body* in its exploitation of the monologue form to probe Watkins' painful personal history, characterized as it is by stigma and marginalization. Both performers liken themselves to Christ, using their suffering as a tool to disseminate some of the harms still inflicted on queer-identified individuals and HIV-positive people.

Unlike the quasi-utopian and apparently community-building prophetic figure that Miller embodies through intense audience interaction, however, Watkins' oblique humor, arcane cultural references, and indirect mode of address distance him from spectators. As one reviewer of Watkins' performance at the Adelaide Fringe put it,

> There was a disconnect between audience members and between the audience and Watkins, and the gaps between these spaces increased with every lonely, hesitant laugh.
>
> *The Year of Magical Wanking* is a series of deeply personal tales, interesting stories performed with skill. What the barrier between me and the performance was I don't know. (Howard 2012)

The effects of this distance unsettle aforementioned links between solo performance, testimony, and an imagined queer community. As we will see, Watkins consequently rejects the tacit deal that other crowdfunded HIV/AIDS playwrights tend to strike with their benefactors – a deal in which a solo performer's saleable persona goes some way to addressing a crisis of knowledge surrounding HIV/AIDS and, therefore, fulfills the funder's philanthropic desires.

To start untangling the political dimensions of Watkins' mode of indirect audience address, I turn to the play's prologue:

> Great Spirit and Great Mystery hear my prayer.
> Bless all the beings gathered in this room.
> I bid your tastebuds welcome to my womb.
> This is my truth. I bare my fruit. Let's share [...]
> I am Neil Martin Watkins and I am
> A sex and love addicted innocent.
> There's patterns I've adopted that would taint the
> Love of Saints. I wank, therefore I slam. (Watkins 2012, 293)

Although not explicitly stated, the 'Great Spirit' and 'Great Mystery' Watkins describes could well refer to the translated names of a deity known as Wakan Tanka in Native North American Sioux tradition, particularly considering his later references to two-spirited people, a designation used in Indigenous communities to describe those who fulfill a traditional third gender role beyond those of man or woman.

Wakan Tanka is thought to be the creator god by the Sioux: rather than embodying a personal god as in monotheistic religions, this supreme being represents an all-encompassing essence that is present in every being and object, thereby resembling aspects of pantheistic and animistic beliefs (Leeming 2006, 399). That Watkins invokes this esoteric spiritual presence at the very beginning of *TYoMW* immediately alerts us to his unorthodox approach to the relationship between performer and spectator. Rather than conceptualizing the audience as a boundaried entity comprised of self-governing individuals, Watkins entreats an amorphous and all-encompassing spiritual essence to hear his stories. The non-specificity of this audience unsettles the intimate nature of the traditional testimonial form: by addressing anything and everything, Watkins refuses to acknowledge the spectators as comprising their own small 'community' as Heddon, Román, or Hughes might have it.

By labeling the work a piece of slam poetry, Watkins even reformulates the performer–spectator relationship's conventionally pedagogical edge. As Susan Somers-Willett explains, poetry slams are not constructed around the same social norms and politesse associated with traditional readings. Rather, the attentional onus is placed on the poet, who 'should compel the audience to listen to him or her' (Somers-Willett 2009, 5). Slam poetry frees audience members from traditional spectatorial obligations, subverting the notion of the testimonial form as something through which performers disseminate vital knowledge and allowing spectators to judge the esthetic value of poetry regardless of their individual credentials or expertise. In subscribing to its tenets, Watkins signals that he is not interested in the solo form as a means to disseminate incontestable truths regarding the experiences of individuals marginalized by hegemonic powers. Rather, as demonstrated by his prefacing the show with a 'prayer', Watkins seeks guidance and knowledge about the *conditions* of his marginalization, particularly regarding matters of bodily autonomy. From the play's outset, it is clear that *TYoMW* does not represent a community-building queer political project in the tradition of, say, Hughes or Miller, who, instead of asking questions, use their platforms to denounce marginalizing hegemonic forces while necessarily participating in neoliberal institutions. Watkins appears to be less willing even than Hoyle to accept the neoliberal bureaucracy of such institutions as a necessary evil. Rather, he tacitly questions the political efficacy of what has become a traditional form of queer testimonial theater.

Albeit Watkins resists reaching out to an imagined queer community via testimonial forms, he still has much to say about the notion of community more generally and its relationship to himself as a queer-identified and HIV-positive individual (and, of course, to the forces of neoliberal hegemony). Without diverging too far from my exploration of HIV/AIDS theater's funding structures, I turn to *TYoMW*'s exploration of the complex links between national and sexual shame and Ireland's precarious post-2008 economy to support Miranda Joseph's theories surrounding 'romantic' communities discussed in Chapter 2. Such links will clarify Watkins' reluctance to treat the audience as its own communal entity and his willingness to approach crowdfunding in a riskier way than other contemporary HIV/AIDS playwrights, using his platform to highlight capitalism's assault on HIV-positive people.

As Joseph explains in a chapter on the discourses of what she terms global/localization, 'Even as capital (and information and people) flows ever more unfettered across the boundaries of nations, traveling great distances instantaneously, capitalism, we are told, attends ever more precisely to place and culture and depends ever more profoundly on the extra-economic bonds of community and kinship' (Joseph 2002, 147). She identifies an increased emphasis on the importance of 'the local' in globalization discourse that can be synonymized with the popularization of neoliberal community discourse. Like 'community', 'the local' invokes 'particularity of identity, social relationships, and values against the abstraction of capital' (Joseph 2002, 147). Localization discourse is also vulnerable to hegemonic neoliberal influences. Much of Joseph's chapter explores parallels between the notions of kinship, community, family, and nationalism, and the ways in which they are variously deployed to bolster a distinctly neoliberal agenda and sell the fiction that, in a world of globalized markets, cultural group formations can exist while remaining untouched by the influences of capital. In idealizing the local as a necessary adjunct to the success of globalization, dominant powers offer a neat and seductive (if unevidenced) solution to people's yearning for community as a counter to alienation. Of course, this solution provides 'too perfect an answer [... and] once again constitute[s] community as autonomous from capitalism and modernity' (Joseph 2002, 152). By dealing explicitly and frequently with the fact of his own Irishness in *TYoMW*, therefore, Watkins is well placed to explore the extent to which local narratives are affected by the workings of neoliberal hegemony.

In the context of Watkins' upbringing, the complicated links between an imagined Irish Catholic community and capitalistic structures are clearly tangible in his (sometimes contradictory) articulations of shame. Watkins' monologue is peppered with questions, both rhetorical and implicit, about the shame he feels surrounding his experiences of sexual abuse as a young boy, his own sexual desires, and, of course, his HIV diagnosis. He asks, for example, in response to the tears shed while thinking of past abuses,

> What's with this flood?
> It's been locked up inside of me so long.
> It isn't right to interfere. It's wrong.
> I don't know why I'm crying. For my blood. (Watkins 2012, 310)

The dimensions of Watkins' shame are shown here to be very complex. While his tears appear at first to represent a response to memories of being abused as a child, he later attributes them to his HIV-positive blood, illustrating the ways in which the roots of trauma can be entangled and impervious to anatomization.

Both HIV and sexual abuse are invasive, capable of crossing borders both physical and imaginary and, as demonstrated by the euphemistic language used to describe trauma (abuse becomes 'interference' while his seropositivity becomes merely 'blood'), the source of indignities he is unwilling to engage with or fully accept. That he claims not to know why he is crying is evidence of disorientation or dissociation designed either to fool himself or his audience into believing he is unscathed by the past, as well as acknowledgment of the multidimensional, interdependent origins of shame. Later in the play, however, despite the obvious difficulty of disentangling shameful feelings, Watkins opens up to the idea of confronting his pain directly. Initial feelings of denial are sharply contrasted by the first few lines of a section entitled 'June':

> I don't know many people who were not
> Abused. That's just being Irish. Forty shades
> Of shame. We all submit when men invade.
> Rape is the culture that we know. (Watkins 2012, 316)

By attributing his childhood abuse to the simple fact of his Irishness, Watkins reformulates and metaphorizes personal pain into a collective national trauma that, as evidenced by the turn to more forthright terminology surrounding rape and invasion, he is less keen to cover up.

This metaphor is consonant in some ways with what Josep M. Armengol identifies as an established political tradition in Irish poetry to personify Ireland as a defenseless woman vulnerable to rape and violation by an English invader, most notably in the aisling genre developed in the seventeenth and eighteenth centuries (Armengol

2001, 8). Feminizing Irishness in this way reflects at once what was seen as Ireland's shamefully subordinate position in Anglo-Irish colonial history and, as Armengol explains, the strength of a kind of nationalism which 'transformed Irish women into "living" representations of the myth of the Motherland', sullied victims of a rapacious England intent on ruining Irish culture (Armengol 2001, 11). More recently in Ireland's poetical canon, this notion was famously addressed and deconstructed in Seamus Heaney's poem 'Act of Union' (1975), which refers, of course, to the 1801 Act of Union that served to merge Ireland and Great Britain into a unified state for over a century. In it, Ireland is figured as a once-ravished, now long-suffering mother whose 'stretchmarked body' must endure 'big pain/ That leaves you raw, like opened ground, again' (Heaney 2001, 24–8). Watkins' conflation of his shame and vulnerability with Irishness, therefore, suggests that the shame that he (and, indeed, others) have endured at the hands of individual men cannot be disentangled from the (gendered) collective shame brought about by a long history of perceived failures by the nation state. While Watkins refers most obviously here to the multitude of historical sexual abuse scandals to have come out of Ireland and its Catholic Church in recent years, the feeling of shame that runs throughout *TYoMW* can thus also be traced back to political and cultural forces that extend far beyond the country's religious institutions alone.

For instance, beyond the intimate details of Watkins' life, this question of shame and bodily autonomy might be read as synecdochal of the wider economic autonomy of Ireland following the collapse of the so-called Celtic Tiger and the accompanying articulations of national shame. The Celtic Tiger era can broadly be described as the period between the mid-1990s and the late 2000s during which the Republic of Ireland experienced unprecedented economic growth, before falling deeply into recession around the time of the global financial crisis of 2008. As Marcus Free and Clare Scully note in an essay on shame and confession in the context of post-Celtic Tiger Irish media, a distinctly neoliberal discourse of somatic self-discipline and control arose in response to the economic crisis that somehow spoke to 'a learned predisposition towards habitual and corporal modesty and self-regulation peculiar to Irish Catholicism' (Free and Scully 2018, 309). As the country struggled under the weight of national debt, its government rolled out austerity measures that placed responsibility for the economic downturn on individuals, a strategy Colin Coulter characterizes as a means to protect the interests of a wealthy few. In official discourse, he notes, 'the origins of the crash are often located in a certain presumed pathology among the Irish people. Retrospective accounts of the Celtic Tiger period are often replete with the language of lunacy', with high-profile figures casting the borrowing boom that fueled the crisis as a form of madness, rather than an inevitable corollary of financialization (Coulter 2015, 10–11)

The reality, of course, is multilayered and complex. On top of an increase in spending and borrowing across Ireland, the boom years are traceable to a variety of interlinked governmental factors such as corporation tax cuts, relatively recent access to trade in the European Union, and a raft of new industrial policies. Pathologizing the Irish citizenry, therefore, was a politically expedient way to protect and support the neoliberal status quo by placing the burden of guilt on individuals, forcing them to 'atone' for previous consumer choices through an austerity program that saw deep cuts to public services. In this way, Free and Scully argue, 'the articulation of a post-boom shame was indicative of how neoliberalism became intertwined with an equally specific and deeply ingrained Irish Catholic culture of self-denial as morally uplifting and a means of atoning for guilt' (Free and Scully 2018, 309). The disorientation and shame expressed in the previous passage, therefore, represent Watkins' personal inability to conform to such ascetic dictates, an apparent failing he frequently connects to both his seropositivity and sex and drug addictions. As well as committing a variety of sins that flouted the expectations of his Irish Catholic community, Watkins fails to adhere to a distinctly neoliberal ethics of self-care and personal responsibility.

This link between religious and neoliberal asceticism is exemplified well in the 'December' section of the play, in which the consequences of Watkins' lack of self-discipline under the neoliberal hegemony are made clear:

> It is a council flat where I reside.
> Since I confessed to having HIV
> My family all agree it should be me
> Who holds the fort for Grandad who's just died.
> Somehow the Council buy he's still alive.
> No legal right have I to warm his bed.
> But I sure need a place to rest my head.
> I couldn't just inherit it. I lie […]
> The Council after two years have copped this
> And wish for me to leave. It's time to go.
> I'm shocked. This is so sudden. I don't know
> Where I'll end up. I fear the street's abyss. (Watkins 2012, 298)

Watkins' family's decision to place him in a risky housing situation as a consequence of his seropositivity is clearly punishment for a perceived inability to maintain control of his health and finances. Rather than support him in their homes and take on the burden of 'shame' related to his HIV diagnosis and welfare needs, Watkins' family pushes him into a council-owned flat he is not entitled to inhabit, effectively leaving him at the mercy of an increasingly frugal state. Reading this passage alongside Joseph's work gives us an insight into how Watkins deconstructs the so-called 'fetishization of family—our ability to forget that our attachments to our families are economic' as well as its wider links to the 'romantic' conceptualization of community and kinship constructed by neoliberal hegemony (Joseph 2002, 165). As Joseph explains, citing work from ethnographer Sylvia Yanagisako, kinship relations serve to arrange and concretize economic hierarchies even in economically prosperous states. As Yanagisako's study of Italian family firms showed, the ideologies of kinship that structured the management and ownership of the firms represent complex processes that serve to both punish and protect members of a given network, depending on how well they fulfill their roles as generators of capital or participants in social reproduction (Joseph 2002, 159). As a productive entity under capitalism, then, Watkins' family is bound to some extent by the productivity and ability of its members to fashion a disciplined and 'sellable' self – exemplified, perhaps, by the uplifting instances of empowerment and self-salvation experienced by Kitchener and Hall's protagonists.

Read in the context of post-2008 economic precarity in Ireland, Watkins' plight is symbolic of wider issues surrounding a similarly circumscribed 'local community' under post-Celtic Tiger Irish governance. The description of Dublin's streets as an 'abyss' – somewhere devoid of human care or interaction – symbolizes the decimation of the welfare state under austerity and the privatization of care into the hands of families and similar kinship structures. In this way, Cormac O'Brien notes, Watkins

> performs the fears of an increasingly disenfranchised working- and middle-class made precarious by an ever-escalating programme of economic austerity. Coupled with this is his search for some meaning and pride in an Irishness that is no longer completely its own master, an Irishness now tainted with the shame of non-sovereignty, and that particularly stigma-inducing troika of the EU, the IMF, and ECB. Watkins's performance is thus imbued with and informed by the powerlessness of the quotidian Irish experience that operates outside

> of, and is yet moulded and shaped by, political and economic forces beyond its control. (O'Brien 2013, 82)

In this way, Watkins draws parallels between his feelings of personal shame and exclusion from the family unit, and a more generalized 'Irish shame' and exclusion from the local community. As Coulter notes, Ireland's economic crisis in 2008 generated a discourse of communality and collectivity that centered on sacrifice and financial expiation (Coulter 2015, 15). Access to this community, however, was dependent on an individual's ability to remain financially independent and not reliant on state welfare provisions. Consistent with neoliberalism's atomizing function, Watkins' seropositivity, financial troubles, and sex and drug addictions (all of which signal an inability to atone for various kinds of 'shame' through self-regulation and asceticism) exclude him from a multiplicity of kinship groups and communities.

Parallels between these romantic conceptualizations of Irishness and the caring family unit also extend to the notion of queer kinship and community. Rather than conceptualize HIV-positivity as something around which queer communal ties can be nurtured, Watkins consistently portrays his serostatus as a barrier to making affective connections with others. This is best articulated during moments when he describes attempts to hook up with other gay men in Dublin:

> I used to be good looking. But who cares.
> I'll die soon with some luck. Won't have to face
> Up to the years I've put on weight. My waist
> Is fine. It keeps the predators in their
> Apartments. Out of mine. Can't give them AIDS.
> I call it AIDS sometimes. I know I'm fine.
> I shouldn't have told anyone. To thine
> Own self be false and to them all. Display
> A milky mask of cow manure and moo.
> Why can't I just get on with life? There's queers
> Are riddled years and they seem grand. It's fear
> That keeps me locked inside my rut. I know.
> I watch the real boys pick each other up.
> I am the last of the great gay ashamed. (Watkins 2012, 316–17)

By describing potential sexual partners as 'predators', Watkins laments what he sees as the anti-communitarian culture propagated by other gay men in the city. As in Lachlan Philpott's *Bison*, Watkins conceptualizes this culture as dependent on the logic of commerce. As an overweight man whose good looks have apparently faded, Watkins views his lack of success with other men as a product of his 'unsellable' body and inability to adhere to the self-regulatory principles that could increase the 'value' of his person.

Clearly connected to the unmarketability of his appearance is Watkins' shame surrounding his HIV diagnosis. By erroneously describing himself as having AIDS – a condition that generally develops when the HIV virus is not treated and controlled with antiretroviral drugs – Watkins gestures toward feelings of lost somatic autonomy or self-control. Within this framework, his virus is an undesirable attribute that could endanger the so-called 'real boys' of the sexual marketplace (the 'market players', perhaps) and is connected to an apparent inability to practice self-discipline and adhere to the neoliberal tenets of self-betterment and growth. Again, therefore, Watkins' feelings about his HIV status represent one element within a complex nexus of shame involving his Irishness, his place within a neoliberal family-oriented society, and his connections to other gay men in the city. Like Joseph, Watkins is suspicious of the overlapping notions of kinship, family, community, and 'the local', albeit in less explicit terms. As a consequence of this resistance (or, perhaps, failure) to submit to an atomistic neoliberal politics, his past experiences are replete with instances of exclusion from every one of these group entities.

Having established Watkins' misgivings surrounding the notions of (queer) community, kinship, family, and 'the local' – all of which he implicitly suggests are polluted by the touch of neoliberal ideology – I will return to the ways in which the performer uses the (cost-effective) solo form to interrogate such notions. Again, Greer's *Queer Exceptions* offers a helpful framework through which to examine such a complex solo performance as *TYoMW*. While Greer frames Hoyle as a 'pariah', he conceptualizes Watkins as a 'martyr' figure. The martyr solo performer, Greer claims, allows us to examine the conditions under which politicized subjects are permitted – urged, even – to voice the concerns of a certain identity group, however broad. Despite neoliberal hegemony's insistence on responsibility and self-regulation, the martyr presents 'the possibilities of endurance as a mode of resistance and self-definition which operates through "the vulnerability and incapacities of the body rather than its prowess"' (Greer 2018, 52). Although Watkins appears vulnerable, then, describing a series of ways in which he has been let down, harmed, or even attacked throughout *TYoMW* – and while he might not boast a body that is traditionally powerful or desirable – his presence as the central and only figure on stage represents a kind of strength and autonomy that allows him to survive without depending on the financial or social structures of neoliberal hegemony.

As Greer puts it, this kind of exceptionalism, while necessarily perpetuating some of the hegemonic configurations of power, also manifests and makes clear 'neoliberalism's incompleteness and inconsistency in a manner that manifests the possibility of resistance, critique and change' (Greer 2018, 51). As already discussed, the inconsistencies that *TYoMW* exposes are detectable in neoliberal configurations of collective groups such as communities, nations, or kinship structures, and the solo form facilitates the exposure of inconsistencies by extricating the 'martyr' from complicity with the individualist and corporatist structures of such groups. This extrication is achieved, Greer argues, through the adoption of 'a mode of truth-telling which extends beyond the singularly exceptional body or circumstances of the performer to become available as the site of communal identification and feeling' (Greer 2018, 77). As O'Brien puts it, 'Watkins's performance is an act of transference, shifting shame back onto the socio-political and cultural structures in Irish life that stigmatise the HIV-positive body in an effort to control it' (O'Brien 2013, 81). Rather than simply expressing his shame as the product of a series of circumstances exclusive to him and others within an imagined 'community' of other HIV-positive people, Watkins identifies the ideological structures that conspire to marginalize and subjugate a multiplicity of identity groups. Instead of using his shame as a means to turn his audience into a 'community' through empathetic identification of similar kinds of personal shame, Watkins reconceptualizes shame as something immanent to neoliberal articulations of community, nation, or kinship that categorize people in order to control them.

In this way, Watkins uses solo performance to upend traditional modes of testimonial theater and to deconstruct 'romantic' articulations of community, while still opening up a space for audiences to consider areas of communal identification. Rather than building a community with distinct boundaries by acting as a 'surrogate' for the experiences of a particular identity group, these communal identifications (seropositivity, for example, or Irishness and its '40 shades of shame') are means to uncover long-standing mechanisms of oppression naturalized by neoliberal hegemony. By denaturalizing such mechanisms through a narrative of exceptional endurance, Watkins calls out to anyone and everyone (the 'Great Spirit' referred to earlier) to look critically at the ways in which neoliberal forces have conspired to push him out of structures of care into economic precarity, and to recognize the ways in which the same thing could potentially happen to others. While, like Hoyle, he does not offer any specific solutions to this issue, particularly in relation to HIV stigmatization, his refusal to adopt the traditional calls for community that tend to accompany testimonial solo performance lays the foundation for a politics resembling something that Jeremy Gilbert terms a 'politics of the common' as opposed to a neoliberal politics of community.

By reconfiguring the necessarily exclusionary language of community as a language accessible to all members of society – the commons – Gilbert argues that the mechanisms of marginalization exemplified by Watkins (and conceptualized as a political impasse by Hoyle) can begin to be tackled. Distinct from the idea of community, the commons do not require participants to share identities, bonds of kinship, or cultural norms. Rather, 'they will be related primarily by their shared interest in defending or producing a set of common resources, and this shared interest is likely to be the basis for an egalitarian and potentially democratic set of social relationships' (Gilbert 2015, 165). Watkins' open audience address at the beginning of *TYoMW* is an example of commons-based discourse. It elides the individualism that might inhere in community formations and, by extension, fights their hierarchical tendencies and exclusionary mechanisms. Rather than positioning himself as a pedagogical figure in the tradition of testimonial solo performance, therefore, Watkins simply opens up opportunities for spectators to identify areas of common experience that shine a light on the harm neoliberalism inflicts on a wide range of subjects, potentially energizing a politics that is not merely contained within a specific (queer) community. That Watkins makes no explicit calls to action, however, reflects an inability or unwillingness to envision concrete counterhegemonic strategies beyond the auditorium. Like Hoyle, there is a sense of political paralysis in *TYoMW* in its inability to reconcile Watkins' counterhegemonic politics with his involvement in the neoliberal theater institution. Despite the lack of a coherent way forward, however, it is abundantly clear that Watkins' solo performance lays the groundwork for a queer politics that is cognizant of the ways in which the oppression and stigma experienced by people with HIV are tied in with the marginalization of a range of other identity groups that fail to assimilate within a neoliberal heteronorm.

To conclude this chapter, therefore, I draw attention to Watkins' deeply personal reaction to achieving his funding target. As the note of gratitude on his Fund It page (an Irish crowdfunding website) reads:

> The value of art in society is that in this case it can help relieve the despair. The audience feels less of an outsider and more part of a

> shared experience. *We are all outsiders* in one way or another. And its [*sic*] not always easy to secure financial aid for work that holds such an extremely outside perspective. Especially in a show about chronic masturbation to S&M Porn. Now in my world that should fill every seat. But we're all different I guess. My name is Neil Watkins and I'm addicted to making theatre. Thanks for enabling me. (Mc 2011, emphasis mine)

The passage strikes a bittersweet note, doing away with the optimistic view of theater as playing a functional role in 'solving' problems like the HIV/AIDS crisis, addiction, or societal inequality, and turning instead to its ability to bond 'outsiders' together in solidarity. In so doing, Watkins demonstrates that the aforementioned capitalistic elements inherent in the crowdfunding model are not totalizing. Rather, as with any counterhegemonic move, artists must participate in the distributive structures available to obtain the resources necessary for producing art allowing them to undermine such structures. In 'reliev[ing] the despair' and producing shared experiences and understandings, Watkins' play helps lay the foundations for the commons we need to alter social relations and improve systems of care.

CHAPTER SIX

HIV/AIDS Theater and Progressive Neoliberalism

In the penultimate scene of Kushner's *Angels*, Harper recounts her dreams while on a night flight to San Francisco. Describing a vision in which souls of the dead rise through the sky to repair the ozone layer, she explains: 'Nothing's lost forever. In this world, there is a kind of painful progress. Longing for what we've left behind, and dreaming ahead' (Kushner [1993] 2017, 285). This bittersweet note of optimism pushes back against what the play's eponymous Angel diagnoses as humanity's addiction to movement and change: 'In *YOU* the Virus of TIME began! YOU *Think*. And You *IMAGINE*! *Migrate! Explore* –' (Kushner [1993] 2017, 169). The pandemic times through which the play's characters live throws this conflict between movement and stasis into sharp relief, as Prior's AIDS diagnosis and quickly weakening body force him to question whether 'progress' can ever accurately describe the changes that affect a society perennially beleaguered by pain and death. Belize, meanwhile, adopts a straightforward if fatalistic attitude toward progress, noting that Prior is 'afraid of … of what's coming. Afraid of time. But see that's just not how it goes. The world doesn't spin backwards' (Kushner [1993] 2017, 175).

As explained in the first chapter of this book, questions surrounding the meaning and value of progress are enmeshed within *Angels*' political and philosophical foundations, inspired as it is by Walter Benjamin's 'Theses on the Philosophy of History'. This essay, penned in 1940 while Benjamin lived under constant threat of capture by Nazi forces, rejects historicist notions of linear progress, invoking the image of Paul Klee's painting *Angelus Novus* to make a case for reconsidering how we think about the past in relation to the present and its politics. Kushner's Angel represents an obvious allusion to

Benjamin's description of the Angel in Klee's painting, whose 'face is turned towards the past. Where we perceive a chain of events, he sees one single catastrophe which keeps piling wreckage upon wreckage and hurls it in front of his feet' (Benjamin [1968] 2015, 249). Benjamin figured the job of the historical materialist to identify 'the signs of a Messianic cessation of happening, or, put differently, a revolutionary chance in the fight for the oppressed past. He takes cognizance of it in order to blast a specific era out of the homogeneous course of history' and in so doing 'blast open the continuum of history' (Benjamin [1968] 2015, 254). Historical moments must not be consigned to a timeline – and thus considered irrelevant to the present moment – but should remain in dialectical tension with current and future-oriented politics. While Benjamin refers here, of course, to the need to reconsider a kind of bourgeois historicism in the struggle against fascism in the 1930s and 1940s, Kushner repurposes this argument to suit 1980s' America. In what ways, he asks, does the HIV/AIDS crisis undermine the foundations of what society has come to accept as progress? And what hegemonic narratives course through our everyday lives – virtually unnoticed – as a means to distract us from the dark underbelly of US capitalism and imperial domination?

One would be hard pressed to find other HIV/AIDS plays that contain *Angels'* philosophical commitment to the interrogation of societal progress, beholden as many playwrights are to 'commonsensical' notions of what advancement looks like. Since the neoliberal turn, the hegemonic conception of progress appears to have centered around two key ideas: 1) progress as measured by heuristic markers of economic growth, such as gross domestic product (GDP), and 2) progress as measured by society's general treatment of historically marginalized groups. On both measures, a superficial glance at the evidence could suggest positive signs of improvement and movement toward kinder and more prosperous societies, at least in the Global North. The volume of global GDP has almost quadrupled since the 1980s (Armstrong 2022), while an increasing number of women, ethnic minority, and LGBTQ+ individuals have secured high-ranking and well-paying positions in public life in countries like the US and UK, thanks in part to the mainstreaming of equality, diversity, and inclusion (EDI) frameworks across public, private, and third sector institutions.

One would be forgiven for presuming, therefore, that the combination of rising overall wealth and increasing representation for minority groups would serve to enhance social mobility and nurture the so-called meritocracy of which free market fundamentalists dream.

The reality on the ground, however, betrays a much less rosy situation for everyone but already-wealthy asset holders. As Grace Blakely sets out in *Stolen: How to Save the World from Financialisation* (2019), a critique of the capitalist economy's latest neoliberal incarnation, financialization's legitimacy relies on the fiction of trickle-down economics, in which entrepreneurs reinvest their profits for the good of the many:

> Whilst all capitalist systems are premised upon the monopolisation of the gains of growth by the people who own the assets, under finance-led growth these dynamics become more extreme. Rising private debt might conceal this fact during the upswing of the economic cycle, but when the downturn hits it becomes clear that finance-led growth is based on trickle-up economics, in which the gains of the wealthy come directly at the expense of ordinary people. (Blakely 2019, 14)

Neoliberalism's representational politics embody similar trickle-down myths to its economic politics. Increased representation for marginalized groups in elite spaces should, so the story goes, break down prejudicial attitudes among the wider public and create new opportunities for young, minoritized people to enter high-ranking and better-paying careers. Pitted against the stark realities of 'trickle-up' economics, however, the vast majority of people in minoritized groups have remained at the peripheries of economic and social life. In the US, for example, extreme wealth disparities between Black and white Americans have barely budged over the past seventy years (Mineo 2021), while wealth disparities between single women and single men are actually widening (Ceron 2023).

Neoliberalism has – at least until recently – successfully maintained consent for such injustices by hammering trickle-down fairy tales into its citizenry, a strategy Nancy Fraser terms 'progressive neoliberalism'. While it might sound oxymoronic, progressive neoliberalism represents a somewhat concessionary formulation originally designed to assuage widespread discontent with the brazen social illiberalism – or 'reactionary neoliberalism' – of the Reagan era. As Fraser explains, 'only when decked out as progressive could a deeply regressive political economy become the dynamic center of a new hegemonic bloc', particularly in the US, where 'common sense was still shaped by New Deal thinking, the "rights revolution," and a slew of social movements from the New Left' (Fraser 2019, 13). Progressive neoliberalism satisfied popular cravings for fairness and social diversity by shrouding deeply regressive financial structures in emancipatory ideals of empowerment, environmentalism, and multiculturalism. The emergence of a seemingly more egalitarian form of capitalism gave neoliberal policies and principles a new forward-thinking and socially liberal gloss, helping to keep questions about capitalism's expropriative underbelly at bay. As such, 'policies that fostered a vast upward redistribution of wealth and income acquired the patina of legitimacy', and the financialization of the economy was allowed to run riot (Fraser 2019, 14). While progressive neoliberalism quietly squeezed precious drops of wealth from everyday workers, the increased availability of financial products and the promise of prosperity to come quelled the possibility of dissent and warped class consciousness. Even the fallout from the 2008 financial crash failed to make serious inroads into cracking this hegemonic bloc. As Fraser notes, the presidency of Barack Obama shored up consent for the status quo by employing a hopeful rhetoric of change and 'recovery', while relying on Wall Street to clean up the mess of the economy and perpetuate the capacities of the elite to hoover up wealth from below (Fraser 2019, 19).

Drawing our attention back to HIV/AIDS theater, progressive neoliberalism's ability to turn heads toward an optimistic future played a crucial role in crafting the public-health-oriented work explored in previous chapters. Perhaps inevitably, these contemporary plays adopt a formula that lends itself well to the sophistic teleology of progressive neoliberal ideology. The 'progress' which many such plays hope to support occurs at the level of individual thought and self-betterment – toward a future in which rational thought and an educated public operate as the ultimate prophylaxes against HIV transmission. Just as hard work and capitulation to free-market diktats represent a boon to economic prosperity in progressive neoliberal logic, such *seemingly* simple and rational behaviors become the ultimate salve for decades of death and illness. To clarify, my critique of progress is not to deny that a future free from HIV is attainable. If we follow a logic of anti-capitalist critique in which use-value takes precedence over the alienating degradations of exchange-value, it becomes clear that tackling the pandemic requires as many intellectual and material resources as we can afford. However, when confronted with the profit-making exigencies of the capitalist mode of production, such an urgent approach would inevitably vex the common sense of our era.

Beyond its institutional manifestations, progressive neoliberalism's decrepit model of societal advancement has gently crept into those subaltern communities it works to marginalize. As explored in previous chapters, the romance of community has often worked to cushion the effects of capitalist dispossession on minoritized constituencies and offset the possibility of counterhegemonic dissent.

However, beyond such deterrent effects, progressive neoliberalism has gone one step further in securing its hegemonic integrity and shaping the definition and function of 'queer' in its own image. This chapter examines a strand of HIV/AIDS theater that buys into a politics of 'queer heritage', in which the gay or queer-identified lay claim to a narratively coherent and collective history – largely built around stories of overcoming the so-called 'crisis years'. This narrative apotheosizes individual activists and freedom fighters as instrumental in softening attitudes toward certain forms of queerness, while providing a blueprint for future generations to live freer lives and pursue their deep-rooted goals – 'progress', in other words.

I contend that while such generationalism is seductive in its promise to construct bright futures from an injured past, it necessarily utilizes an essentialist rhetoric of kinship and quasi-familial bonding that precludes the solidaristic politics necessary to confront neoliberalism's cruelties. By presenting the formation of contemporary queer identity as a frictionless movement toward a coherent goal, generationalist narratives shroud the spiky political terrain that accompanies such a broad identificatory constituency. While a wealthy, gay, cisgender man in Manhattan might share the queer identifier with a Black, unhoused, transgender woman living in Detroit, for example, their respective material interests and relation to the neoliberal state are wildly different. Neoliberal common sense that touts the vitality of finance capital and the sound morality of individuality will, inevitably, appear more convincing to our well-off New Yorker, whose specific embodiment of queerness does not preclude wealth, respect, and assimilation. In other words, the extent to which queer individuals are subject to exploitative behaviors, state neglect, violence, and stigmatizing practices tends to shape their politics, leaving plenty of scope for discord and intracommunity struggle. As Gilbert and Williams note, 'All political constituencies are multiplicities, and the task of radical politics is always to create material, organizational, and cultural conditions under which the progressive potentialities of those constituencies will be expressed, while their reactionary potentialities will not. The war of position is over potentialities' (Gilbert and Williams 2022, 88). Building on this Gramscian insight, any queer movement committed to improving the material conditions of those who contravene sexual modernity's conjugal imperatives and gender binary must show potential beneficiaries of such norms how they stand to lose out as a result of neoliberalism's other exploitative and alienating functions. Generationalism fails in this regard. Rather than clarify the role of, say, marriage in providing the material conditions and social reproductive labor capitalism requires to thrive, generationalism uncritically celebrates such forms of kinship and conceptualizes the struggle against oppression as a battle of symbols and ideas alone.

As we will see, generationalism's inadequacies are becoming especially clear in the early to mid-2020s – a moment in which progressive neoliberalism's fundamental contradictions are emerging from the shadows. While progressive neoliberalism remains influential across much of the corporate and governmental spheres, worsening living conditions, international tensions, and the looming threat of climate change are laying the groundwork for waves of counterhegemonic action and the splintering of community formations. For example, while progressive neoliberal orthodoxy has been touting LGBTQ+ acceptance (albeit contingent) for several years, queer individuals are facing renewed threats from the reactionary right as the 2020s progress, with transgender individuals bearing the brunt of moral panics and exclusionary state policies. At the same time, such panics are nudging the political 'center' rightwards, casting transgender women as a threat to social cohesion and fracturing ties between variously marginalized groups under the queer umbrella. We are – as Gramsci so famously put it – living through an 'interregnum' (Gramsci 2003, 276).

Theorized as the moment in which a tired hegemonic order has almost broken down and society awaits the emergence of fresh ideological configurations, an interregnum offers only murky glimpses of the future. Even renowned political theorists appear to scramble in the dark for clues to humanity's next move, offering significantly divergent views about the prospects of such hefty concepts as capitalism, democracy, liberalism, and more. Fraser views 'progressive populism as the likeliest candidate for a new counterhegemonic bloc. Combining egalitarian redistribution with nonhierarchical recognition, this option has at least a fighting chance of uniting the whole working class' (Fraser 2019, 30). Wendy Brown, meanwhile, argues that democratic principles have atrophied to such an extent under neoliberalism that society is growing increasingly vulnerable to plutocratic and quasi-fascistic political forms. 'Instead of being politically pacified', she explains, 'citizenries have become vulnerable to demagogic nationalistic mobilization decrying limited state sovereignty and supranational facilitation of global competition and capital accumulation' (Brown 2019, 84). Regardless of one's view about neoliberalism's likely fate, however, the political limitations of generationalism are abundantly clear when we consider how hegemonic blocs have treated various forms of sexuality as means to uphold their dominance.

As Christopher Chitty explains, sexuality has been molded and shaped throughout history as a means to control the forces of production and statecraft:

> The problem of sexual hegemony is both a question of establishing whether same-sex attraction, solidarity, and erotic attachments as such presented particular relations of force within an antagonism that required neutralization; and a question of what relations of force in a particular conjuncture enabled the repression of same-sex attraction, solidarity, and erotic attachments or, conversely, allowed them to exist unperturbed. (Chitty 2020, 172)

As we careen into uncharted conjunctural waters, in which hard-won rights might be expediently sacrificed for hegemonic means, I question the political sense of generationalist rhetoric. In relying on teleological and highly partial accounts of queer identity development, it underestimates the potential antagonisms within and between different expressions of queerness, and fails to appreciate the counterhegemonic work required to continue fighting repressive sexual regimes. As I will explain through analysis of two generational HIV/AIDS plays – Matthew Lopez's *The Inheritance* (2018) and Damien Atkins, Andrew Kushnir, and Paul Dunn's *The Gay Heritage Project* (2013) – some of the most popular contemporary HIV/AIDS plays appear unfit to broach the political questions of our current conjuncture and present questions about what a genuinely counterhegemonic theater might look like.

Third Way neoliberalism in Matthew Lopez's *The Inheritance*

By far the most notable and critically lauded example of generational HIV/AIDS theater is Matthew Lopez's *The Inheritance,* which premièred at London's Young Vic Theatre in 2018, directed by Stephen Daldry. Written in an American context, it creatively reimagines E.M. Forster's novel *Howards End* (1910) as a means to explore the intergenerational dynamics existing among a large group of gay men living in New York in 2016, as well as to question how their lives have been shaped by gay men of the past, Forster included. Forster appears onstage as Morgan, an almost spectral presence who helps Eric and Toby (the play's central couple) and their contemporaries to narrativize accounts of their young lives. Perhaps inevitably, *The Inheritance* focuses heavily on the ways in which the AIDS-related deaths of many gay men in the 1980s and 1990s have affected gay and queer-identified youths in the twenty-first century, particularly in regard to their sense of identity and understanding of queer history, activism, and HIV-positivity in the present. This is done primarily through Walter, an older character who describes his experiences of the early decades of the epidemic in detail to Eric, encouraging the younger man to imagine how such a crisis would affect his life were it to happen today and to address a supposed generational amnesia surrounding AIDS. Tied in with this, however, are broader-reaching questions about how an increasingly capitalistic political economy has affected the possibility of a queer heritage. Unlike many of the contemporary plays discussed in this study, *The Inheritance* features explicit and extensive discussion between its characters about contemporary political issues, touching on topics including Donald Trump's election, spiraling levels of poverty and financial inequality in the US, and the ways in which these topics intersect with queer politics.

In Daldry's production, many such conversations take place around a large, raised platform, generating scenes reminiscent of an academic roundtable. During these scenes, the young men relay their thoughts about the evils of the Republican Party and the culture of self-interest they detect within its heart, alluding sometimes to the rise of President Trump and his legislative actions. Nowhere is this more starkly demonstrated than during a heated discussion between Henry Wilcox, one of the play's older gay men who is both a millionaire businessman and a donor to the Republican Party, and a group of younger gay men with Democratic leanings. After accusing Henry of forgiving the Reagan administration's inaction during the early years of the AIDS crisis, Jasper, one of his younger peers, exclaims: 'Your party is presently attempting to ram through Congress a bill that would strip twenty-three million people of their health insurance just so that you can have another tax cut that you don't need' (Lopez 2018, 169). Here, he clearly denounces Trump's aim to dismantle the Patient Protection and Affordable Care Act, a federal statute designed to minimize the number of Americans without medical insurance. This kind of anti-free-market discourse runs throughout many of the conversations that take place around the table, something that has not gone unnoticed by *The Inheritance*'s many reviewers. Neil Dowden, for example, notes the play's interest in exploring 'collective responsibility versus individual freedom, and idealistic bohemianism versus materialistic capitalism' (Dowden 2018). Writing for *Variety*, meanwhile, Matt Trueman states that '[l]ike *Angels in America, The Inheritance* [...] is a vast, imperfect and unwieldy masterpiece that unpicks queer politics and neoliberal economics anew', even going on to decree that the play 'is, above all, a damning indictment of individualism; the play's every relationship effectively an economic arrangement, prostitutes and kept husbands alike' (Trueman 2018).

As we will see, however, such analysis of the play overlooks how its characters' progressive economic critiques belie their investment in neoliberal common sense, which infiltrates spheres seemingly unrelated to political economy. As Doreen Massey noted in conversation with Stuart Hall, burgeoning political crises (like the Trumpian healthcare plans condemned by Jasper) should be thought of

> as complex moments, where different parts of the overall social formation may themselves, independently, be in crisis in various ways, but at a certain point they are condensed. Although we see this moment as a big economic crisis, it is also a philosophical and political crisis in some ways – or it could be, if we got hold of the narrative. So it's really important that we don't only 'do the economy', as it were. (Hall and Massey 2010, 59)

Although Massey is referring to the rise of neoliberalism in the British context, her emphasis on looking beyond the realms of the economic to understand major political and social changes is vital for any study of the function of hegemony. While Jasper might offer economic arguments that go against the hegemonic grain, the way in which he and his contemporaries discuss the notion of heritage is often markedly homonormative. Even as the unions of convenience discussed by Trueman might indeed be read as indictments of the exploitative or self-serving impulses generated by neoliberalism, most are broken up by the end of the play, replaced by conventionally 'healthy' monogamous relationships that emulate those seen in first-generation HIV/AIDS plays. Characterized as the means by which to build a 'cherished family home', live a life 'filled with love' and, for one character, as an apparent 'salvation' from sex work (Lopez 2018, 294), such unions make coherent a call for queer generationalism that mirrors familial bonds traditionally associated with the heteronorm and supported by neoliberal hegemony.

Somewhat ironically, underlying this appropriation of the ideal family unit is an attempt to counter the recrudescence of regressive and fascistic attitudes in the US in the 2010s and beyond. In a bid to hold on to the rights their forebears helped secure, the men in *The Inheritance* rummage through queer history to find lessons applicable to the present day. Speaking to director Stephen Daldry, a writer for *The New Yorker* explains:

> addressing contemporary politics offered opportunities for exploring how the activism of the past might inform the present. "People had come to accept the idea that rights were rights," Daldry told me. "And what we understand now is that they can be taken away from you really easily. 'Act up, fight back' is not a slogan from the eighties and nineties—it's an active slogan that we need now." (Mead 2019)

Here, Daldry imagines a coherent genealogy that begins with ACT UP's counterhegemonic actions and leads directly to the fight against Donald Trump. Although highly conscious of the potential for cultural regression surrounding sexual liberties, Daldry embraces teleology by placing his faith in imagined queer epistemologies. What this approach overlooks is the extent to which queer liberation has relied on the shifting material exigencies of the ruling class. As Chitty's study emphasizes, histories of sexuality have often narrativized sexual intolerance as the result of regressive religious and moral ideologies. However, while it is tempting to celebrate the gradual breakdown of binary sexual regimes as evidence of an enlightened society, analyzing the wider political and economic systems within which sexual norms emerge can reveal double-edged implications.

As Sita Balani notes, in consonance with Chitty's central insight, relatively recent shifts in queer acceptance were implemented at least in part to fulfill decidedly less liberatory goals. Balani takes as an example the neoliberal 'Third Way' of the 1990s, a (seemingly) more socially liberal hegemonic bloc best encapsulated by the governance of Tony Blair in the UK and Bill Clinton in the US. Following Blair's victory in 1997, New Labour implemented a raft of policies that brought the lives of gay people in line with those of heterosexuals, including the equalization of the age of consent and the introduction of civil partnerships. Such changes reflected the exigencies of a globalized and financialized world, as 'New Labour saw homophobia as an outdated stigma that prevented gays from realizing their potential as full economic actors and citizens of the nation' (Balani 2023, 82). In clearing the path for a productive and financially liberated gay constituency, however, New Labour inevitably took aim at new targets deemed unable to contribute to societal 'progress'. Tasked with generating a citizenry capable of driving productivity and growth, 'New Labour focussed their attention on an "underclass" which they characterised as feckless and work-shy, living in dysfunctional families, unable or unwilling to embrace the promise of sexual modernity' (Balani 2023, 89). Sexual practices and norms were considered integral to the development of productive workers, with phenomena such as teenage pregnancy, casual sexual encounters, single parentage, and early marriage lumped together as an affront to the integrity of neoliberal capitalism. As Balani's central thesis convincingly elucidates, such practices were often stigmatized along racial lines. Pakistani and Bangladeshi communities, for example, 'were viewed as adhering to the "old-fashioned" pattern of family formation, with early marriage and childbirth as a norm, while Caribbean communities [were] placed as their polar opposites, as having chaotic domestic lives without coherent family units' – both representing threats to neoliberalism's new ideal of the double-earner family (Balani 2023, 91).

Similarly stigmatizing and racializing norms embedded themselves into Bill Clinton's version of the Third Way. As Fraser notes, Clinton's administration bears a 'heavy share of responsibility for the weakening of unions, the decline of real wages, the increasing precarity of work, and the rise of the "two-earner family" in place of the defunct family wage' (Fraser 2017b, 42). Marrying traditional welfare statism with Reaganite economics, Clinton's Third Way is best typified by the Personal Responsibility and Work Opportunity Reconciliation Act of 1996, which, as he explained in an announcement on the legislation, sought to give people 'a chance to draw a paycheck, not a welfare check' through a series of cuts to welfare provisions (*The New York Times* 1996). The bill was shot through with a markedly neoliberal emphasis on personal responsibility, with the President explaining that it 'must not let anyone off the hook [...] We have to make sure that in the coming years, reform and change actually result in moving people from welfare to work. The business community must provide greater private-sector jobs' (*The New York Times* 1996). While rejecting the Reagan administration's explicitly demonizing, often racist rhetoric surrounding people in receipt of help from the state, Clinton tacitly cast welfare claimants as undeserving freeloaders. Given the fact that benefits were largely routed to those who fell outside of the double-waged family unit, Clinton thereby managed to demonize queer and racialized minorities via a more circuitous route.

So, Daldry's faith in the idea that 'rights were rights' reflects a somewhat parochial attitude that fails to appreciate neoliberalism's reliance on the continued production of exclusionary norms and stigmatizing practices. In so doing, it flattens the dynamism of 'progress' to a tussle between the 'good' (progressive) and 'evil' (reactionary) sides of neoliberal party politics. During one of the play's many roundtable discussions, for example, a character known as Jason 1 talks about the inequalities queer people face in contemporary America, imploring his peers to 'talk about suicide, violence, homelessness. These are the things that will require just as much of our attention as marriage equality did and these are the things we have the chance to make some real progress on once [Hillary] Clinton is elected' (Lopez 2018, 85). Here, Jason displays a materialist's awareness of the ways in which injustices largely considered to be class-based – such as homelessness – are inextricably entwined with the oppression of queer constituencies. However, his uncritical confidence in the Democratic presidential candidate, a feeling reiterated over and over again by many of the play's young gay men, demonstrates faith in a two-party system whose participants largely differ in their bluster and rhetoric, rather than the material effects of their policies.

Of course, to read the young men's unshakeable support of Hillary Clinton as airtight evidence of the play's underlying political project or message would be rather facile. The men's verbal sparring matches with Henry at times expose logical flaws on both sides of their arguments, and even serve to encourage feelings of sympathy toward the older man. When discussing how Henry made his millions, for example, Jasper states: 'For a man like you, being gay is just a speed bump on your journey. You've arrived at your station in life without ever once understanding suffering or the meaning of adversity' (Lopez 2018, 171). This touches a nerve in Henry, prompting an uncharacteristically emotional outburst about the pain and fear he experienced during the height of the AIDS crisis in the 1980s and 1990s. Jasper, meanwhile, is made to seem closed-minded, even unduly cruel in his presumptuous verbal attacks. In some ways, then, *The Inheritance* can be seen to reveal the deficiencies of the dual-party system of allegiances that has structured the US political landscape for decades and encouraged both sides to generate false or reductive presumptions about one another, denting their capacities for reasoned discussion.

The liberal Forsterian basis on which the play is built, however, does not blame these communication problems on the severely limited political horizons of two-party politics. Rather, it couches the problem in idealist, hegemonic terms, asserted most concisely in a phrase uttered by Margaret Schlegel in *Howards End* – 'only connect'. When Margaret wants to challenge the conservative and unmerciful views of Henry Wilcox (on whom Lopez's Henry is based), she decides to 'only point out the salvation that was latent in his own soul, and in the soul of every man. Only connect! That was the whole of her sermon. Only connect the prose and the passion, and both will be exalted, and human love will be seen at its highest' (Forster [1910] 2012, 195). Such passion, for Margaret, in a liberal humanist sense, is to be found in the beauty of art and cultural productions and, more broadly, in the spirit of social connection. She believes that to reconcile his conservative economic rationalisms, Henry must realize the passionate love that lies latent within him and, supposedly, every person. Lopez's Henry, then, remaining somewhat true to his literary namesake, also becomes conscious of such passion when pushed to consider the pain of losing precious friends to the AIDS crisis. Cross-generational bonding, the play implies, is a means to rebuild lost social connections, reignite Henry's passion, and allow the gay men to work together across the party-political divide toward a better future free from oppression.

Look beyond the content of *The Inheritance* itself to the material aspects surrounding its production, however, and this claim to political nuance appears to sit on shaky ground. If potential audience members were in any doubt as to the political bent of those involved with the play's production, they need only turn to its official Facebook page to observe obsequious posts dedicated to the former presidential nominee. One of the images posted on the page, for example, in which actor Kyle Harris appears wearing a T-shirt emblazoned with the campaign slogan 'I'm With Her', reads 'Happy Birthday, Hillary Clinton! Jasper (Kyle Harris) is with you now and forever' (The Inheritance Play 2019a). This sentiment is similar in tone to references made by the young men about Clinton in *The Inheritance* itself and serves as evidence of its underlying ideology. Tristan, for example, exclaims 'My girl's gonna win!' (Lopez 2018, 86) during one of the play's political discussions, while a scene involving the 2016 election results sees the young men don 'I'm With Her' garments and wave campaign flags supportive of the Democratic candidate. In so doing, the group apotheosize Clinton as a quasi-matriarchal symbol of their politics and demonstrate their allegiance to progressive neoliberalism.

In some ways, the strength of this allegiance can be read as Hillary Clinton's consecration into what D. Gilson conceptualizes as a kind of neoliberal 'divahood'. Gilson argues that the rise of neoliberalism over the twenty-first century has seen more traditionally defined gay icons or 'divas' such as Whitney Houston or Cher increasingly replaced by figures like Clinton, who straddle 'the line between pop icon and political powerhouse' (Gilson 2015, 627). Noting that women who reach divahood status are typically required to earn it by turning public tragedy into triumph, Gilson essentially argues that the criteria for 'triumph' in an increasingly corporatist world are being modified. Once thought of as a woman who necessarily overcomes public humiliation to find her talents blossoming in the music industry or in Hollywood, the diva might now simply embody what Fraser terms 'a meritocratic corporate feminism focused on "leaning in" and "cracking the glass ceiling"' (Fraser 2017b, 42). As Gilson explains, 'the social mobility of diva-ed celebrities [is comparable] to the "competitive, self-interested individuals" of the emergent political condition' (Gilson 2015, 62). Clinton's trajectory from First Lady of the United States – a subordinated and historically gendered role – to the winner of the Democratic nomination in 2016 might be read by her fanbase as evidence of her unique ability to overcome obstacles and win power. It should be noted, of course, that the consecration of female celebrities and political figures as divas is multidimensional: it is a complex process that a number of scholars have attempted to unravel through psychoanalytic theory and queer theories exploring the performative dimensions of camp. Ultimately, as Edward R. O'Neill explains in an essay considering the cultural logic of the diva, 'Gay men and divas, fags and femme fatales: we are bound together by a logic we yet dimly understand' (O'Neill 2007, 11). For the purposes of this study, however, it is useful to observe the willingness of Clinton's queer fanbase to deify her as the archetypal self-made woman and symbol of 'meritocratic' modern feminism, despite the obvious fact that her political powers have been boosted by ties to her husband. That Clinton is 'diva-ed' in similar ways to gay icons of the past, I argue, evidences the ability of neoliberal common sense to invade and capture virtually all cultural phenomena.

It could be argued, of course, that the young men's fervent support of Clinton is borne of an urgent desire to avoid a Trump-led administration at any cost. In a political environment where neoliberalism can degrade and immobilize leftist movements relatively easily through the seductions of corporatist common sense, progressive neoliberalism might *appear* as the most viable weapon against its more reactionary incarnations. As remarked in *The New Yorker*, '*The Inheritance* [...] raises alarms about the potential reversal of the legal advances that have been made in L.G.B.T.Q. rights. Audience members of any age or sexual orientation may feel a nightmare being replayed when, in Part 1, the friends gather to watch the 2016 election returns' (Mead 2019). In other words, Trump represents the ultimate nightmare that must be countered by the election of Clinton, the only other electoral candidate with a chance of taking office. As explained in the introduction to this study, the Trump administration has made legislative moves regarding HIV/AIDS policy that threaten the wellbeing of HIV-positive and queer-identified people. It has also made moves to dismantle LGBT rights across a number of areas beyond healthcare. As an article for the *Guardian* stated in September 2019, '[s]ince taking office, the Trump administration has sought to reverse healthcare protections for trans people, moved to ban trans people from serving in the military, eliminated rules protecting trans students and pushed to allow businesses to turn away gay and trans customers if they seek a religious exemption' (Levin 2019). Such vociferous and remorseless attacks are, of course, in line with the reactionary neoliberalism Fraser conceptualizes, and exemplify why the young men in *The Inheritance* attach themselves so fervently to the progressive neoliberalism offered by Hillary Clinton.

The ways in which this attachment relates to anxieties surrounding Trump are best exemplified by a diatribe against Henry's decision to contribute to the President's campaign fund launched by Tristan, a young HIV-positive physician:

> If America is a body, then that man you gave money to is HIV: an opportunistic infection that has invaded a compromised nation at its cellular level and that is now destroying its ability to defend itself by replicating its genetic material from person to person, across the entire nation. HIV may be treated at the cellular level, but it affects the entire body. And individuals alone cannot cure what ails this country. It requires a community response. (Lopez 2018, 168)

It should be noted, first of all, that Tristan's extended metaphor does not quite work here. HIV is not, in fact, an opportunistic infection. Rather, it is a retrovirus that weakens the immune system and renders an infected person increasingly more susceptible to opportunistic infections that would not otherwise have made them ill. Disregard this relatively minor misconception, however, and the metaphor clearly reveals something of how Tristan makes sense of the Trump phenomenon and the era of reactionary populism through which he is currently living.

The notion that individuals are made into Trump supporters and sympathizers via the replication of genetic material suggests that they comprise their own community unit bounded by quasi-familial bonds. In some ways, this idea parallels the kinship structures of the men in the play, who frequently espouse neoliberal notions surrounding duty, family, and the privatization of care. As the official website for *The Inheritance* states in bold letters on its homepage, the play represents an examination of 'how much we owe to those who lived and loved before us, and questions the role we must play for future generations' (The Inheritance Play n.d.), particularly considering the ways in which reactionary neoliberalism threatens to eviscerate the rights older queer people worked so hard to secure. In conceptualizing both groups as delimited by kinship – as warring families, perhaps – the young men make sense of the contemporary political moment via identitarian forms of politics, somewhat insensible of the ways in which class concerns and neoliberalism's track record of immiserating poorer echelons of society laid the groundwork for Trump's election victory.

To clarify, figuring Trump alone as the malignant pathogen behind the rise of reactionary neoliberalism is to ignore the ways in which previous administrations – including those headed by Democrats – have executed a slew of neoliberal policies that siphoned both money and power into the hands of the already-wealthy and away from poorer members of the citizenry. To metaphorize Trump-voting US citizens as diseased or infected situates the misogyny, racism, and homophobia espoused by the President within their very cells, essentializing the Trump voter as passively susceptible to opportunistic malignancies. In marking themselves out as members of the 'disease-free community', the young men conceptualize the idea of political affiliation not as a complex and ongoing process of grappling with hegemonizing forces and one's material conditions, but as a simple case of intrinsic identity. By splitting the citizenry into the 'infected' and the 'healthy', Tristan's metaphor embodies a reductive and destructive notion that Trump voters are irredeemable 'deplorables', born with racism, homophobia, and misogyny in their blood. While some progressives might hold this view, reactionary populists are just as prone to distorted forms of thought, reinforcing the view that 'all progressives are incorrigible moralizers and smug elitists who look down on them while sipping lattes and raking in the bucks' (Fraser 2017a). Such beliefs reveal a misdirection of anger and grief toward citizens who do not hold the capital or levers of power required to improve everyday people's lives – the result, no doubt, of hegemony's uncanny ability to distract from its root inequities.

Of course, the HIV metaphor in some ways absolves Trump supporters of responsibility for their reactionary political views. By pathologizing their allegiances in such a way, Tristan portrays them as helpless victims whose capacity to comprehend the common sense of progressive neoliberal hegemony has been injured. Trumpism has rid them of their rational minds, and they require 'community' to mobilize and cure them of their ailments. This notion is in some ways redolent of what Fraser identifies as 'progressive moralism' in some factions of the neoliberal establishment, 'which routinely portrays [rural Trump voters devastated by unemployment] as culturally backward. Rejecting globalization, Trump voters also repudiated the liberal cosmopolitanism identified with it' (Fraser 2017b, 43).

Anxieties surrounding so-called 'high culture' and the importance of being 'cultured' (particularly within the circles of metropolitan gay men) course throughout *The Inheritance*. Although Trump-sympathizing Henry's extraordinary wealth sets him apart from the rural voters to whom Fraser refers, he appears similarly plagued by an aversion to the kinds of artwork, films, and literature around which Eric and his friends center much of their lives, making broad comments such as 'I find most contemporary fiction glib and self-conscious' (Lopez 2018, 116). When Henry and Eric's relationship starts to blossom, Eric makes it his mission to expose Henry to cultural products that he believes will 'broaden [the] horizons' of his older friend. As one of the young narrators goes on to explain, 'Henry's life was entrenched completely in commerce. Yet in the weeks that followed, Henry spent more time inside theaters, museums, and concert halls than he had in decades' (Lopez 2018, 117). Here, commerce and culture are seen as somehow antithetical, despite their obviously tight-knit relationship. This is, again, a moment in which Lopez's attachment to a Forsterian imperative to 'only connect the prose and the passion' – realms distant from the rational economic – is made clear. Henry's engagement with the world of business and his desire to accrue wealth have apparently injured his capacities to enjoy the cultural wares New York has to offer and, by extension, extricated him from a community of cultured gay men of which all of the other characters seem to be a part. Like his namesake in Forster's novel, who sees civilization as 'moulded by great impersonal forces' (Forster [1910] 2012, 200), Henry must ignite unrealized artistic 'passion' to become a more 'feeling' person within the constraints of neoliberal hegemony by enjoying choice cultural products.

In Eric's mind, his identity as a gay man is intrinsically tied to the realms of art and culture. When contemplating the ways in which HIV/AIDS has potentially affected the notion of gay heritage, for example, 'Eric wondered what his life would be like if he had not been robbed of a generation of mentors, of poets, of friends and, perhaps even lovers' (Lopez 2018, 147). By nestling the word 'poets' in among more general modes of relation such as 'friends' and 'lovers', Eric grieves for what he sees as the unusually brilliant – and now forever untapped – artistic talents of a generation of gay men. While it could easily be true that scores of gifted young poets died of AIDS, Eric's decision to bemoan the collective loss of artistry over other forms of talent appears to essentialize gay men as natural purveyors of high culture. Eric is oblivious, of course, to the fact that his socio-economic position has provided access to virtually unlimited cultural products and therefore influenced his artistic proclivities. At the beginning of the play, for example, Morgan describes how, 'through no enterprise of their own, [Eric and Toby] were the inhabitants of an enormous three-bedroom, two-bathroom apartment with a terrace' that Eric took over after his grandmother died (Lopez 2018, 11). The couple talk of having scant finances yet appear to live lives of relative luxury: Toby can afford to dedicate his life to writing while Eric relays his plans for a season of theatergoing and attending film festivals without appearing to lend a second thought to the costs.

The men's social circle is also confidently *au fait* with the vernacular and conventions of certain cultural institutions, evidenced, for example, when Adam describes how he 'grabbed a rush-ticket spur of the moment' for a ballet recital (Lopez 2018, 36). The use of the word 'grabbed' here, evocative of a rough or snatching movement, reveals Adam's entitled attitude toward his own spectatorship at cultural events: the option to attend the ballet is simply there for the taking, as and when the mood arises. Furthermore, while rush-tickets might offer cheaper ticket prices than those booked in advance, they also require buyers to familiarize themselves with the operative conventions of individual theaters, such as when and where to queue up or call for tickets, the dates and times of productions, and, of course, whether last-minute tickets are offered at all. This is where the mentorship that Eric mentions comes in. Throughout the play, Eric is preoccupied with the notion and practice of cultural mentorship between his queer kin, educating Adam about cinema of the French New Wave and Henry about German Expressionism, and, as demonstrated in his grievances regarding HIV/AIDS, contemplating the mentorship of which he himself might have been 'robbed'. This mentorship role is, of course, closely related to that taken on by biological parents in more heteronormative kinship structures, imbued with the privatized 'responsibilities of care' written into the script of neoliberal hegemony.

Despite the obvious ways in which Eric's mentorship role is undergirded by narrow, elitist conceptions of taste and class, the political discourse that runs through *The Inheritance* barely pays heed to how issues surrounding wealth and class might interact with, and produce, different forms of oppression. In neglecting these class dimensions, the young men of the play are impelled to construct a genealogy of queerness that makes sense of past injustices through other relational factors. They look toward the affective bonds that tie generations together – often strengthened by shared wounds inflicted by a distant, pathologized Other – as well as an apparent shared appreciation for cultural products, essentializing the queer subject as somehow blessed with brilliant sensitivities toward high art. In so doing, the play constructs a crude genealogy of queer 'community' pitted against other bounded groups, rather than as a porous and often disjointed genealogy of sociopolitical movements that have countered, and sometimes capitulated to, broader hegemonic structures. It is in this way that the young men's clear adherence to neoliberal doctrine undermines their attempts to address problems surrounding privatization and the further dismantling of welfare provisions in the US in any rigorous way. It is quite clear that the heritage constructed in *The Inheritance* is influenced to some extent by the common sense of progressive neoliberalism and the political exigencies of a Trumpian moment.

Having established the neoliberal capitulations made in Lopez's play, then, the question of whether an anti-neoliberal account of queer heritage could have a place on the mainstream commercial stage remains unanswered. A quick look at the marketing materials used to attract audiences to *The Inheritance*'s Broadway production is enough to reveal the difficulty of such a project, so beholden is the mainstream theatrical institution to the idea that its clientele harbor individualistic proclivities and a kind of hermetic communitarianism. When the play made its transition to the US, for example, a campaign was set up encouraging audience members to, as a rather cryptic campaign video implores, 'Tell us a story' and 'Tell us the story of us, how we got here' (The Inheritance Play 2019b). The play's official website also includes a 'Community' page that states: 'Tell us about a person who has influenced you or your community for the chance to be featured!', encouraging users to fill out a form sharing 'Your Story', name, and Instagram handle (The Inheritance Play n.d.). In some ways, this campaign represents an attempt to cast the play's net beyond the constituency of wealthy New York gay men depicted in the play, encouraging people from a range of backgrounds to fill the auditorium. It also, however, reinforces the boundedness of the notion of community that we have returned to so frequently in this study.

On the one hand, inspiring people to consider the ways in which older generations have paved the way for improved rights and freedoms for certain identity groups serves, in some respects, as an urgent warning to protect their achievements against the rise of reactionary neoliberalism and barely veiled fascistic populism. The urgency of this message could go some way to explaining why so many plays focused on the notion of queer heritage comprise the third generation of HIV/AIDS theater. On the other hand, however, it is important to question how the play operates politically in such volatile times. As one journalist speculates about Tristan's metaphorization of Trump as the HIV virus and his followers as infected cells: 'In London, the tirade elicited applause; on Broadway, it should bring the house down' (Mead 2019). The idea of an auditorium of (largely moneyed) New Yorkers fervidly cheering on Tristan's assertions that isolate the pathological, tainted 'communities' or 'cells' from the cultured, healthy ones is, I argue, deeply troubling in that it appears to celebrate the political 'purity' and righteousness of those in the room, thus obscuring how the material conditions created by neoliberal legislation might have created such a divide in the first place. It is an image that destabilizes the notion that affective bonding alone, at the expense of a more materialist-oriented political dramaturgy, might effectively work toward a utopian vision of a society free from oppression, particularly in the profoundly divided climate of Trumpian America.

The Gay Heritage Project: historicizing queerdom onstage

By way of comparison, we turn to a play that attempts explicitly to address some of the problematic aspects of queer heritage that Lopez's play avoids. *The Gay Heritage Project* is a quasi-documentary play following three gay men as they conduct research into a complex question: whether they can claim a form of alternative gay heritage that stands outside that of the conventionally familial. As a play that dedicates itself to establishing whether such a thing as queer generationalism even exists, *TGHP* is interested in unraveling how the evolution of queer politics has been tightly entwined with that of capitalism over the latter half of the twentieth century and beginning of the twenty-first. Combining the disparate dramaturgical traditions of documentary theater, autobiographical testimony, farce, and magical realism, *TGHP* features scenes spanning a range of localities and eras as a means not only to reflect on the personal histories and experiences of its creators (known in the aggregate as the Gay Heritage Project Collective), but to investigate how far these experiences correspond with those of other queer people around the world, both past and present. While HIV/AIDS is not necessarily the overarching theme of the play, it makes several appearances as a contingent theme in the trajectory of queer history.

In an introduction to the play, one of *TGHP*'s writers, Andrew Kushnir, states that he and his collaborators – Damien Atkins and Paul Dunn – figured themselves as 'creator-performer-investigators working in and with community' when coming up with its central concept (Kushnir et al. 2018, xiv). Rather than figuring 'heritage' as a coherent and singularly defined entity, they embraced it as an action: 'an exchange, a theme party, a social rite' (Kushnir et al. 2018, xvii). In an introductory section of the published playtext entitled 'What is Heritage?', the collective explains that 'Heritage is, or should be, the subject of active public reflection, debate, and discussion. What is worth saving? What can we, or should we, forget? What memories can we enjoy, regret, or learn from? Who owns "The Past" and who is entitled to speak for past generations?' (Kushnir et al. 2018, xxiii). This sentiment represents a call to collectively probe the politics of historicizing queer history. Rather than offering concrete conclusions, the play simply represents the continuation of, as writer Atkins puts it, 'a conversation that existed before we came along, that we enjoyed sharing with an audience' (Kushnir et al. 2018, xxi).

However, while the impulse to interrogate the notion of queer heritage is by no means novel, the play's creators are keen to foreground their awareness that the emergence of gay, lesbian, and queer identities is a relatively recent phenomenon. Any quixotic notion that this triumvirate of gay male playwrights could establish a neat and narratively coherent genealogy of similarly identified gay male forebears – E.M. Forster, for example – is quickly put to rest. Citing John D'Emilio's seminal essay 'Capitalism and Gay Identity' and David Halperin's 'Is There a History of Sexuality?' as influential research materials for *TGHP*, Kushnir explains in the playtext's introduction that the GHP Collective were forced to relinquish certain romantic notions of a queer past as soon as their investigative project commenced. Kushnir describes the sense of disappointment and even grief that he and his fellow writers felt when confronted with theoretical materials that challenged the 'pride and sense of lineage invoked by things like Ned's speech in Larry Kramer's *The Normal Heart*', in which a long list of writers and philosophers from Aristotle and Socrates to James Baldwin and Herman Melville are posited as powerful determinants of queer culture (Kushnir et al. 2018, xv). Of course, as D'Emilio's essay evidences, the emergence of queer identities should not be so simplistically reduced to a product spawned by the work of a select few. Rather, it must be

> associated with the relations of capitalism; it has been the historical development of capitalism – more specifically, its free labor system

> – that has allowed large numbers of men and women in the late twentieth century to call themselves gay, to see themselves as part of a community of similar men and women, and to organize politically on the basis of that identity. (D'Emilio 1993, 468)

D'Emilio claims that the increasing expansion of wage labor and the decline of household production throughout nineteenth-century America (and, of course, beyond) shifted the meaning of the family from a self-sufficient unit in which every member took on different forms of productive labor, and birthing offspring was seen as an economic necessity, to one which nurtured individual satisfaction and happiness. Releasing individuals from their dependence on the household in this way, D'Emilio argues, supported the separation of sexuality from procreative obligations, creating conditions 'that allow some men and women to organize a personal life around their erotic/emotional attraction to their own sex' (D'Emilio 1993, 470).

Although capitalism helped clear a path toward queer political organization and emancipatory legislation across much of the world, it also nurtured homonormativity, shoehorning non-normative relationships into heterosexist and patriarchal frameworks serving neoliberal ends. The free market fundamentalism undergirding contemporary neoliberal hegemony cannot be untethered from its reliance on a privatized labor force grounded in family and community structures that Peter Drucker claims 'maintain and perpetuate male domination of women, heteronormativity and other inequitable social relations' (Drucker 2015, 340). So, if the queer Marxist texts to which *TGHP*'s creators are 'indebted' and have 'connected with over the years' (Kushnir et al. 2018, 157) are as persuasive and pivotal as stated, analysis of the play should, theoretically, reveal an awareness of what D'Emilio delineates as the dialectic at the heart of capitalism: the 'constant interplay between exploitation and some measure of autonomy' that assures queer people of their increasing freedoms while tacitly curtailing their powers to live beyond the normative kinship structures that sustain neoliberal hegemony (D'Emilio 1993, 468).

A mere glance at the playtext's bibliography reveals the collective's inclination to probe this dialectic: texts cited include D'Emilio's aforementioned essay, Lisa Duggan's 'The New Homonormativity, The Sexual Politics of Neoliberalism' (2002), and Cindy Patton's *Inventing AIDS* (1990), to name but a few. Although not all 31 listed texts are explicitly Marxist or, indeed, would fit comfortably into the category of queer Marxism, most draw lines between capitalistic structures and contemporary articulations of queer sexuality. The GHP Collective's (somewhat reluctant) gravitation toward historical materialism is charted in the first two acts of the play. The first act, entitled 'Can you describe what it is you're searching for?', serves to dispel some of the romantic interpretations of contemporary queerness harbored by *TGHP*'s writers. In one scene, Kushnir searches the annals of the Toronto Public Library to find information about homosexuality in Ukraine. His efforts are, however, in vain, and he is disappointed to discover that his Ukrainian mother's statement that 'There were no people like you where we came from. There's no such thing as a gay Ukrainian' – a reaction to his coming out – appears to be corroborated by the library's material lacunae (Kushnir et al. 2018, 15). The scene, then, offers the first indication that the word 'gay' is not a term appropriate for universal use, whether in terms of region, time period, or any other situational variable.

This realization is made most clearly and comically manifest in the final scene of the first act, a so-called 'image ballet' of 'gays in history'. The stage directions stipulate that the 'ballet' take the form of music-accompanied image projections featuring, firstly,

> *two ancient Egyptians having anal sex. It is the onset of a barrage as more and more images appear, moving ahead in history, until the entire playing area (screen and floor) erupts into a video montage of famous (and some non-famous) gay people, images, and icons from history, bringing us up to the present day.* (Kushnir et al. 2018, 22, italics in original)

While the playtext does not offer concrete suggestions as to which historical figures should be included in the montage, it does feature an exemplary timeline of photographic images and artworks including Peter Paul Rubens' *Saint Sébastien secouru par les anges* from 1604; portraits of both William Shakespeare and Queen Elizabeth I; a daguerreotype of Abraham Lincoln; photographs of Alan Turing, James Baldwin, Barack Obama, and Laverne Cox; and logos for initiatives such as Black Lives Matter and Australian Marriage Equality. By staging this timeline as a 'barrage' of images that fill the entire screen and floor of the stage, an ironic display of ostentatious camp so commonly associated with contemporary gay culture, the notion of gay heritage is shown to be both anachronistic and reductive. Exhibiting such a seemingly disparate array of historical figures whose sexual proclivities varied widely, and many of whom would have been unfamiliar with the semiotics of camp, clearly demonstrates the overgeneralization of 'gay' as a generic term in this context. The montage form itself, meanwhile, is a trope so overused in cinema of the 1980s and 1990s as a means to signify growth, development, and the passing of time (particularly in coming-of-age dramas) that to a twenty-first-century audience it can easily be read as an ironic signifier. The linear simplicity of the 'image ballet' is thus undermined, indicating that the collective is ready to deconstruct its initial notions of gay heritage. Situating this fantastical and comical display at the end of the very first act prepares spectators for a deconstruction of its romantic precepts during the remaining four: once the music has died down, the trio are ready to move on to Act Two: 'Bad News'.

This 'bad news', of course, refers to scholarly theories that the GHP Collective were newly exposed to during their writing of the play. The first scene of the second act takes the form of a farcical imagining of a television broadcast entitled 'The Eternal Gay', a 'program that affirms gay people have always existed, and searches history to uncover gay stories of gay people who are gay', according to its host (Kushnir et al. 2018, 29). The host's repetition of the word 'gay' is clearly intended to undermine the program's lack of historical and intellectual rigor. A character simply known as the Theorist is enlisted to point out the folly of mining history for preconceived conclusions in this way, a method that contravenes the dialectical principles of historical materialism that form the basis of the GHP Collective's research texts. As the theorist notes,

> You're taking modern experience and understanding and reading it backwards in time. It wasn't until decades later, when capitalism and the labour market transformed the function of the family and the structure of society, along with very specific developments in medical and legal discourse, that there was even the availability to assume a gay identity and therefore be a gay person. (Kushnir et al. 2018, 30)

This corrective to the Eternal Gay host's flawed thinking is, of course, redolent of the dialectical approach to history favored by D'Emilio and Drucker and scandalizes the host's stable sense of identity in much the same way as described by Kushnir in the playtext's foreword. 'What happens in the future', the host asks, 'if things continue to change, and we lose this "availability to assume a gay identity"? Could we … disappear?' (Kushnir et al. 2018, 31). The ellipsis in this final question indicates both a sense of shock and an unwillingness to countenance the fundamentally protean nature of queer identity formation in thrall to the tides of prevailing hegemony.

It is in this way that the host represents gay conservatism's resistance to ideas put forward by a certain Marxist vanguard within the field of queer theory. Populated by theorists such as Rosemary Hennessy and, more recently, Peter Drucker, Christopher Chitty, and Holly Lewis, this loose scholarly unit questions the liberatory function of teleological queer politics within a wider anti-neoliberal movement. Hennessy, for example, states that political organization under a queer Marxist rubric requires

> a process of unlearning that opens up the identities we take for granted to the historical conditions that make them possible. It involves uprooting these identities not just from ways of thinking that invite us to construe them as natural but also from a history of suffering – the fertile ground for resentment to grow – and resituating how we know them in a different historical frame, a frame that allows us to see how this suffering is the product of a mode of production that outlaws a whole array of human needs. (Hennessy 1998, 229)

For Drucker, opening up identity in this way is the first step to moving beyond the constraints of the heteronormative family and the ways in which it supports neoliberal tenets. Inspired by ideas put forward by Marxist revolutionary Alexandra Kollontai calling for more open and collective domestic structures, Drucker advocates a queer politics that seeks economic alternatives to the heteronormative family, allowing the security traditionally associated with insular kinship structures to coexist with individual autonomy. He argues that an effective same-sex politics will necessitate a return to the central interests of socialist feminism – namely, social reproduction, family, and gender identity. Such a politics would reveal the fragility of queer people's hard-won rights under capitalism, demonstrating the need for LGBTQ+ advocacy to be 'integrated into a comprehensive programme for reproductive freedom and socialisation of childcare and domestic labour – a programme that would clash with the prerequisites for maintaining profit rates and accumulating capital' (Drucker 2015, 389). In other words, Drucker calls for a fundamental overhaul of the kinship structures supporting the neoliberal imperative for constant and robust economic growth.

At times, *TGHP* demonstrates flickers of a politics implicitly grounded in this drive to renegotiate heteronormative family structures. Most obviously, the writers each offer candid accounts of growing up in family units that treat their identities as discordant and 'unproductive' in some way. Damien, for example, in an analeptic scene that transports the audience back to his childhood in the 1980s, is taunted and teased by his sister and parents for obsessing over figure skating and one of the sport's well-known celebrities, Brian Orser. Searching for some kind of affective connection or role model that he clearly cannot find within traditional kinship structures, Damien abashedly says, 'I don't know. I just feel like ... like he's cool, and like ... maybe it would be fun to hang out because, like, maybe we would have something in common' (Kushnir et al. 2018, 6). The discomfort Damien feels in his family home is palpable, evidenced by dysfluencies in his speech that betray a disorientation in a world that, for a number of imbricated reasons (homophobia, attendant misogyny, and their relations to neoliberal hegemony, to name a few), cannot accommodate his digressions from heteronormative masculinity. Indeed, this familial exclusion is later explicitly articulated and certified by his Uncle Rob, who tells Damien: 'You're not a real Atkins, anyway' (Kushnir et al. 2018, 96).

Andrew, too, who has already had his gay identity muddied by his Ukrainian heritage, finds himself excluded from traditional kinship structures. His mother, he discovers, views this as a necessary evil. She tells a young gay shop assistant from Calgary that his struggles to fit in with the community can be remedied by relocating. When he tells her of his ambitions to work in 'the business side of fashion', she reminds him that 'your life is precious and you only get one. My son is happy, I think. But he had to leave to be who he is. Sometimes you have to leave' (Kushnir et al. 2018, 98). That Paul and Andrew shoot each other a knowing look when the latter's mother describes this encounter is evidence, again, of their discomfort with the coerciveness of heteronormative family structures. As well as pushing queer individuals away from their families, his mother's emphasis on the pursuit of personal happiness (and economic success) reflects neoliberal hegemony's apotheosis of the individual within a market-oriented society built on competition and growth.

Indoctrinated by neoliberal common sense, Andrew's Ukrainian mother has adopted an outlook akin to that of the capitalistic American Dream. So embedded is the corporatist, neoliberal idea of freedom – that is, freedom to participate in markets – that she reduces what must be a painful and difficult decision into a matter of airtight economic logic. Such beliefs, of course, are 'deeply attached to the collective brain stem, which leads to strict acceptance of anything that resonates with the American Dream, even if they are destructive, nondemocratic, or blatantly false' (Magnuson 2018, 158). While Andrew's mother appears to be looking out for the best interests of this young man, her unquestioning acceptance of his need to leave evinces the 'destructive' part of neoliberal hegemony. She views heteronormative family structures as more-or-less fixed units of corporate-minded individuals, each with their own (gendered) roles. As an individual whose identity does not accord with such structures, the man must relinquish affective bonds to achieve his fashion business 'dreams'. In this way, *TGHP* makes clear some of the difficult decisions that queer individuals are faced with when navigating a neoliberal world that ennobles the notion of individual choice and self-sufficiency while simultaneously emphasizing individuals' obligations to the heteronormative family.

Despite the GHP Collective's alertness to, and obvious understanding of, neoliberalism's insidious effects, there are moments when its common sense creeps into the play's rhetoric. This is particularly true of *TGHP*'s paratextual elements which describe its genesis and development. In the section entitled 'Brotherhood', for example, Kushnir describes the play as both 'an expansion of the self', a revolt, and a 'rebellion against the heteronormative hegemony' requiring 'a private renewal, a constant healing of self, a questioning of self, a questioning of loves, a questioning of dreams' (Kushnir et al. 2018, xix). This therapeutic language of healing and renewal speaks to a culture of 'self-care' that, while rooted in radical feminist activism, has been subsumed by neoliberal doctrine. Indeed, 'self-care' serves as a romantic euphemism for the privatization of caring responsibilities, 'obscuring the social, economic and political sources of physical, emotional, and spiritual distress and exhaustion', and underhandedly depoliticizing subordinated groups of people (Michaeli 2017, 53). 'If we are frustrated, sad, or angry', Inna Michaeli notes, 'we mustn't act on it, get angry together, protest and organize for change. The mainstream self-care discourse invites us instead to breath [*sic*], meditate, and – if we can afford it – enjoy a day at the spa' (Michaeli 2017, 53). Kushnir's rallying call here is undermined somewhat by the privatization of caring responsibilities: according to this logic, freeing queer-identified kin (or 'brothers', as the title suggests) from systemic oppression requires transformation and 'work' on an individual level first and foremost. It is no accident that Kushnir's introductory message fails to express the ways in which broader institutions and governmental structures must be overhauled to effect liberatory justice for queer individuals: neoliberal thought ensures that the onus is on individuals themselves.

'Doing' heritage in this way is reflective of something Meg Luxton terms 'perverse individualism' – an individualism that encompasses obligatory caregiving both for oneself and others, as well as competitive impulses. This ideology necessarily divides a citizenry into kinship groups concerned with their own flourishing and economic advancement and is resonant with Margaret Thatcher's often-quoted belief that there is 'no such thing' as society – only individuals and their families. However, while neoliberal hegemony still rests to a large extent on familial structures tied by the twine of biology, Luxton argues that it has had to adapt ideologically in recent years to accommodate the fact that 'most interpersonal relationships, including kin, are increasingly diverse and largely voluntary' (Luxton 2010, 177). One characteristic of this evolution is a valorization of (or simple reliance on) community structures that, like the heteronormative family unit, depend on voluntary caregiving work that lies outside of the labor market.

Certainly, such responsibilities of care abound within *The Inheritance*, exemplified most starkly in the aforementioned cultural mentorship roles adopted by men within its central group of gay male protagonists. However, the rather more diverse queer community Kushnir calls on to fight its own oppression is also shown to be vulnerable to perverse individualism, something best exemplified during moments when the GHP Collective mines the past for activists who had a hand in securing certain freedoms for today's queer-identified contingent. In a scene that imagines the annual general meeting of a group known as the Sissy Liberation Front (a playfully obvious allusion to the Gay Liberation Front), for example, one of the members proclaims:

> Mark my words: each and every one of you is a fucking *soldier*. And the bravest kind. You, like the sissies who came before you, have worn your uniform in your voice, in your hands, in your hips, and you have worn that uniform every day of your life since you were six years old. And thank god for that. Every gay that is, every gay that was, and every gay that ever will be owes you his deepest gratitude. (Kushnir et al. 2018, 123–4)

Such rhetoric is emphatically militaristic. The evocation of gayness as a 'uniform', for example, along with an emphasis on intergenerational gratitude that serves to deify members of the Sissy Liberation Front, is reminiscent of the kind of patriotic rhetoric evinced globally by influential political figures during and after wartime. While, to some extent, such militarism is highly ironic (the reclamation of the derogatory word 'sissy', for example, perhaps serves to undermine historically homophobic military institutions in Canada and beyond), its clear associations with the notion of duty and obligation to one's kin clearly support the privatization of care Kushnir endorses. The apotheosizing of the soldier figure reflects the tenets of perverse individualism in its glorification of military service as the quintessence of competitive triumph and as exemplary of the self-sacrifice required to protect a wider group, buttressing 'a commonsense hegemonic ideology based on the fundamental success of self-actualizing individuals' (Luxton 2010, 180).

To understand why the GHP Collective's self-avowed suspicion of nuclear familial structures seems unfailingly to fall back into subtly exclusionary and, ultimately, neoliberal articulations of queer kinship in *TGHP*, we return again to the notion of 'community'. While the play offers implicit commentary on capitalism's ability to rigidify heteronormative family structures and marginalize the queer-identified, it overlooks some of the ways in which neoliberalism influences broader kinship structures. As already evidenced by *The Inheritance*, community groups are often built around a demographic identifier or shared belief, requiring prospective members to fit certain criteria in order to benefit from the affectively constructed bonds. To some extent, the collective is closely attuned to how the queer community has often been constructed through 'diversity' programs that exploit them as consumer-subjects for profit. Kushnir, for example, bemoans the fact that 'many straight people are not interested in our sensibility beyond its capacity to improve their lives – whether it be through humour, style, aesthetics, reinforcing the sanctity and value and desirability of their institutions. The capitalist machine is interested in us as a niche, as a revenue stream' (Kushnir et al. 2018, xviii). However, this statement is belied by the collective's consistent impulse to grapple for a coherent and bounded queer community within the play.

In the fourth scene of the fourth act, for example, Damien steps aboard a so-called 'Gay Heritage Bus', in which queer-identified people of different races, nationalities, orientations, and genders come together to discuss their differences, because, as he puts it, 'we're all queer – or something in the neighbourhood – and I genuinely feel like *that's* something that connects us...' (Kushnir et al. 2018, 87). Noting that he prefers to spend time in the company of the queer-identified, Damien goes on to say, 'I know there are straight people who would be frustrated by that dividing line just like I'm frustrated by the dividing line between us. But ... I'm here because I'm gay and that's not *nothing*. I know it's not the same thing as race or gender but it's not nothing' (Kushnir et al. 2018, 89). While the theatrical conceit of the bus – a communal and constantly moving space – represents acknowledgment of the fact that societal marginalization cuts across a host of different identity formations, Damien's analytical and political impulse to figure queerness as an identity category whose oppression can be lucidly compared to that of race and gender grates against facets of queer Marxist thought. Indeed, a number of *TGHP*'s source materials foreground the primacy of class analysis in their methodologies and are suspicious of the reification of selfhood that sometimes occurs in identity-based political discourse.

As Barbara Foley argues, the population is necessarily divided up into distinct and ultimately abstract categories in a class-oriented society, ensuring that the productive labor of the many continues to benefit the few. To understand how social inequality works and is perpetuated, therefore, we must investigate how class-based society interacts with categories of identity. While injunctions to explore the role of class in identity formation are sometimes derided as 'class reductionist' (i.e., that which reduces sexism or racism to epiphenomenal categories secondary to class-based oppression), this is not necessarily the case. To include class-based analysis is, rather, 'to insist that the distinction between exploitation and oppression makes possible an understanding of the material roots of oppressions of various kinds' (Foley 2018, 273). While identity-based analysis addresses vital questions surrounding social injustices and inequalities – as Damien rightly notes, these are 'not nothing' – a queer Marxist approach asks us to put such analysis in conversation with broader questions of political economy, with a view to producing more effective forms of counterhegemonic organization.

Such an approach, it has been argued, requires identity groups' relinquishing of investment in an injured past, something that has obvious ramifications for a project on heritage. I gesture most clearly toward Wendy Brown's *States of Injury* (1995) here, which probes the ways in which identity categories are constructed around a sense of woundedness in some examples of leftist discourse. Suspicious of the ways in which politicized identities are articulated against a bourgeois masculinist ideal, Brown claims that the elimination of such an ideal (which, of course, is an implicit aim within marginalized identity groups) requires forfeiting many of their claims to injury and exclusion. While such claims might serve a cathartic or rhetorical purpose in the short term, the idea that they are required 'for the potency and poignancy of their political claims' raises questions about the extent to which 'a critique of capitalism is foreclosed by the current configuration of oppositional politics, and not simply by the "loss of the socialist alternative" or the ostensible "triumph of liberalism" in the global order' (Brown 1995, 61). Theater and performance scholar

Stephen Farrier expresses similar concerns in a paper on intergenerational queer theater, pointing in particular to the fact that plays in this category tend to include somewhat sentimentalized representations of a queer generational gap left by the HIV/AIDS epidemic. Figuring the loss of so many gay men as a wound specific to the queer community, Farrier notes, 'can be damaging because it subtly posits that proper relations between older and younger people are based on kinship models that are cunningly connected to the terms of the heteronormative familial' (Farrier 2015, 1404).

These criticisms ring particularly true during a surreal scene in *TGHP* in which HIV is put on trial in a courtroom. After the character Mr. HIV Virus has been found guilty of one hundred million counts of murder by a character simply known as the Judge, Damien is given the chance to air his grievances against the former. Speaking of his formative years, he explains:

> There was such an *absence*. And I was seventeen – I was vulnerable, and scared, and I needed role models, people to tell me that it was going to be okay, that I could be an out gay man and still be happy and successful and safe. What I needed was a community of elders, of big brothers, but... But as a gay man, I was born into *silence*. (Kushnir et al. 2018, 116)

The character Mr. HIV Virus is, of course, symbolic of the governmental and institutional structures (such as pharmaceutical lobbies) that failed to act on the HIV epidemic during its emergent years, in large part thanks to homophobic/heterosexist stigma. This diatribe, therefore, represents an overtly political attack on the way in which certain lives are valued above others by prevailing heteronormative hegemony. Putting the onus on older gay men as quasi-parental elders to guide him toward 'success', however, paradoxically reinforces heterosexist notions of kinship and heritage by valorizing the forms of voluntary caregiving labor that neoliberalism needs to sustain itself. By investing considerable faith in the notion that bounded community structures can liberate queer-identified people from oppressive powers, Damien is unable to get past the idea that the politics of gay heritage are simply 'not nothing', a double negative aptly reflective of neoliberal hegemony's ability to fold community-based politics in on itself.

Of the two plays, of course, it is clear that *TGHP*'s attempts at a dialectical unearthing of the conceptual history of the gay and queer lend it a more nuanced and coherent anti-capitalist edge than *The*

Inheritance. In it, the collective demonstrates an astute awareness of how articulations of gay and queer identities emerged in a way that is inseparable from the development of capitalism as we know it today. That *TGHP* was staged in a theater that brands itself as exclusively queer while *The Inheritance* emerged on relatively mainstream and financially lucrative stages is no coincidence. Rather, it reflects the demands of the theatrical market broadly speaking: the digestible progressive neoliberalism of *The Inheritance* chimes with a nominally progressive theatergoing public preoccupied with winning a largely symbolic (rather than materially beneficial) battle against a reactionary Other, while *TGHP* is permitted to explore the complexities of queerness, albeit in a way that ends up supporting romantic articulations of communitarian politics. In assessing how *TGHP* finds itself ensnared in neoliberal common sense despite its anti-capitalist theoretical groundings, we can begin to understand why Kushner is so unwilling to disavow or wholly support the notion of progress in *Angels*. While queer generationalism might contain kernels of a utopian countercurrent, its compatibility with progressive neoliberalism renders it vulnerable to hegemonic traps. However, faith in progress *tout court* is surely necessary for an HIV/AIDS theater capable of inspiring positive steps toward a future with greater access to treatments, less stigmatization, and lower rates of transmission. The task for today's HIV/AIDS playwrights is, therefore, to grapple with what progress should look like in a conjuncture where hard-won rights and access to healthcare are all too easily snatched away.

Conclusion: HIV/AIDS Theater in the Era of COVID-19

HIV/AIDS theater has only ever existed in a neoliberal context. Subjected to its individualizing common sense, poorly funded theatrical institutions, and alienating functions, the genre has produced a vast array of works that align with – and grate against – the hegemonic order to varying degrees and diverse political ends. As we have seen, the HIV/AIDS plays that have garnered the highest degree of cultural purchase over the past four decades are those in which an HIV-positive, male, queer subject fights back against homophobic stigma while enjoying some form of assimilation into the dominant culture through, for example, harmonious coupledom. To reiterate the caveats set out in my introduction, plays that fit this restrictive mold do not reflect the broad gamut of HIV/AIDS theater that has graced stages across the anglophone Global North – let alone the wider world. As Alexi Chacon succinctly points out in a recent article about an 'overlooked multitude' of HIV/AIDS plays, those interested in exploring the genre's history will find a plethora of deeply political and experimental works in LGBTQ+ archives and special collections – such as Rhodessa Jones's *Deep in the Night* (1998), a series of monologues focused on Black women's experiences of the virus, or Alberto Antonio Araiza's *H.I. Vato* (1994), which narrativizes the mistreatment of HIV-positive people of color at the hands of healthcare providers (Chacon 2022).

However, that these plays remain tucked away in archives, waiting to be unearthed by those scholars interested in 'fringe' or 'experimental' theater, demonstrates their relative political insularity and limited ability to expand public consciousness surrounding HIV/AIDS. That plays such as *The Normal Heart* return to the stage over and over is not merely down to lack of imagination on the part of artistic directors. Rather, it reveals neoliberalism's unerring ability to pump money into 'safe' or assimilatory theater, strip dissident or visionary artists of the material conditions necessary for survival, and depoliticize the public with whom such artists engage. Since the conjunctural shift toward neoliberal statecraft in the 1980s, we have witnessed a naturalization of individualism designed to convince workers that they are living through a meritocratic era in which people of any race, gender, or sexuality can reap the rewards of the free market. Over the decades, this narrative has chipped away at solidaristic bonds and obscured how the asset-owning classes have hoovered up what little wealth already-exploited communities owned in preceding decades. Under such conditions, the plight of the viral underclass (to use Thrasher's apposite term) has remained invisible to much of the rest of society, while nostalgic histories of heroic overcoming and 'progress' for a delimited queer constituency have crystallized as the overarching story of the HIV pandemic.

Analyzing such invisibilization through a Gramscian lens, society's dominant powers appear to have knowingly aided and abetted the oppression of a viral underclass – at least to some extent. Rejecting the brute economism of more orthodox forms of Marxism, Gramsci posited that 'one consequence of inequalities and hierarchies in power is that those who benefit from them often have the resources to define how everyone's circumstances are interpreted' (Martin 2022, 3). The narrative that HIV/AIDS is no longer a serious problem in the Global North benefits capitalist states by hiding their neglect of constituencies most commonly affected by the virus and, indeed, capitalism's wider inability to generate systems of care that prioritize health and wellbeing over profit. To make this observation is not to diagnose some kind of conspiratorial or premeditative thought on the part of state actors or institutions perpetuating standard narratives about HIV/AIDS. Rather, as the chapters in this book have demonstrated, AIDS nostalgia, individualistic moralism surrounding HIV prevention, and other common-sense notions about the virus are reacting to a wider hegemonic war of position within which we are all entangled.

For example, creating and staging public-health-oriented theater that perpetuates neoliberal diktats about self-preservation and monogamy makes sense within the contemporary theater landscape. The disciplinary functions of 'impact' and profitability requirements, combined with a wider political economy dependent on the subjugation of certain constituencies, serve to create an environment hostile to genuinely counterhegemonic performance work. Most theater makers with a prosocial desire to educate audiences about the virus and reduce transmission rates are bound to mold their political consciousness and artistic endeavors around such requirements, so seductive are the common-sense beliefs peddled by influential forces (particularly those who benefit from these beliefs). Such an observation helps us identify how theater ends up aligning with ideological positions that contradict the interests of the community for which it aims to advocate, and, indeed, those of wider society.

Gramsci's use of military metaphors is, again, instructive here, highlighting the need for new forms of theatrical dissidence that strategically provide subaltern classes with the intellectual tools they need to recognize the terms of their subjugation. For some critics of hegemonic analysis, this abstractly bellicose strategic model is hindered by an authoritarian or statist logic requiring people to ally themselves with a privileged center comprising political thinkers and intellectuals. As James Martin explains, such critics argue that the point of radical politics 'can only be to overcome hegemony. Emancipation today is about subverting the grip of neo-liberal capitalism over every aspect of life, [...] propelled by a militant sense of commitment and a refusal to be captured by power' (Martin 2022, 110). While overcoming the need for such tactical political formations might sound desirable, its idealism elides the impossibility of such a radical epistemological autonomy existing in our current conjuncture. As author Jedediah Purdy writes of his participation in the world of corporate publishing, neoliberal individualism and market-centric values have become so naturalized that 'in a neoliberal world, to act is to accept them [...] The neoliberal public writer can't help being on the market, because the market is what any possible public has become' (Purdy 2014). Our methods of consuming and producing art are so enmeshed within alienating corporate structures and our experiences so shaped by neoliberal logics that dissident political work requires shrewd negotiation with powerful forces, many of which govern the dissemination of cultural products and ideas. While a radical break with the mainstream cultural landscape might seem like an obvious solution to this problem, disengagement from the normative structures that govern our everyday social realities is unlikely to garner the mass support necessary for social change.

With this in mind, what might a counterhegemonic HIV/AIDS theater look like in the 2020s and beyond? As I have indicated, neoliberal tenets are quickly losing their seductive sheen as 'trickle-down' economics reveals its spurious underpinnings. Following the Great Recession, Global North states have (to varying degrees) witnessed growing wealth inequality, social unrest, housing and healthcare crises, incipient authoritarian tendencies, and other morbid symptoms that point toward a hegemon unable to keep a lid on capitalism's spiraling contradictions, as well as a citizenry increasingly unwilling to accept the social structures to which they are beholden. The emergence of COVID-19 is an especially critical moment in this transition from the 'end of history' era to a moment of deep hegemonic crisis. As well as revealing the fragility of healthcare infrastructures bent and twisted out of shape by corporate interests, the virus prompted the imposition of 'lockdowns' around much of the world. Under most lockdown arrangements, so-called 'key workers' – members of the working class fundamental to the running of society such as supermarket staff, nurses, delivery drivers, and bin collectors – were compelled to risk infection and return to work every day. At the same time, members of the professional managerial class were encouraged to work remotely, a privilege made possible by the continued labor of key workers. Quite suddenly, consciousness of our essential interdependence bubbled up among the hemmed-in masses, evidenced by the emergence of mutual aid groups, fulsome attitudes toward key workers, and a generalized sense of social rupture. Or, to put it another way, the pandemic 'made it easier to see oneself more as a node in a biopolitical network to which one is responsible than as an autonomous individual whose sovereignty is guaranteed by free will' (Bratton 2021, 35) – one of neoliberalism's fundamental fictions.

This observation provides a helpful analogue for considering what the future of HIV/AIDS activism, care, discourse, and art might look like as neoliberalism disintegrates. While SARS-CoV-2 and HIV are very different viruses, they share some similarities in their social and political effects. Both affect poor and racialized communities to a greater extent than their white, moneyed counterparts. At the same time, both have played a role in raising class consciousness around the world and precipitating the emergence of urgently political cultural products and discourses. The theater sector, for example – largely demobilized by social distancing rules – quickly ushered its first COVID-19 plays onto the stage as soon as theater doors reopened (often serving significantly depleted audiences). As with much early HIV/AIDS theater, such plays were steeped in the fraught politics of the early pandemic, addressing government mismanagement and the privileging of the economy over people's lives.

In the UK, one of the first and most notable pandemic plays to receive widespread attention was David Hare's *Beat the Devil* (2020), a monologic and autobiographical work about Hare's experience of contracting COVID-19 and suffering severe symptoms. The play's premiere coincided with the reopening of London's Bridge Theatre in 2020, with Ralph Fiennes selected to voice Hare's experiences. Like much of the early testimonial work of the AIDS crisis, such as Miller's *My Queer Body*, Hare's play takes aim at individual figures, rather than systemic capitalist dysfunction. He describes the experience of watching the government's chaotic response as follows:

> Everywhere, as one obscure minister after another stutters and stumbles on the airwaves, people complain that this is a cabinet of mediocrities. But this does violence to the word. Mediocrity suggests middling ability. You and I are mediocrities. These people are incompetents. Ministers like Robert Jenrick, Dominic Raab and Helen Whately, the hapless minister of state for social care, who comes across like a quiz contestant who's forgotten the name of the fourth Beatle – and who is, by the way, in charge of care homes – such people do not begin to merit the word "mediocrity". (Hare 2020, 15)

Of course, the word 'incompetents' absolves minsters like Raab and Jenrick of any moral failing. In contradistinction to Miller's portrayal of Jesse Helms as comedically villainous, these politicians are simply useless at their jobs – the ultimate weakness in a conjuncture characterized by individualism and fantasies of meritocracy. If we dig deeper into the reasons behind such incompetency, however, we start to see its ideological underpinnings. Lack of preparedness, too-late lockdowns, and the outsourcing of crucial healthcare and epidemic control services to private firms such as Deloitte, Serco, and Palantir combined to create a shambolic response that exacerbated the severity of the pandemic. Unwilling to prioritize the citizenry's health and wellbeing over an ideological schema in thrall to the demands of the market, the government 'weakened and fragmented NHS services and local councils' public health departments and undermined the country's ability to respond to COVID-19' (British Medical Association 2020, 2).

Such iniquity is nothing short of what Naomi Klein terms 'disaster capitalism', whereby neoliberal governments exploit public panic and desperation in the midst of crisis to implement radically pro-corporate methods. Typically, this involves pumping government money into private enterprises whose profit-making imperatives preclude the provision of adequate crisis-response services. At the same time, dominant powers obfuscate the ideological dimensions of their actions by branding alternatives options as much less desirable. In overlooking this political chicanery, Hare reveals something of his own class position and alignment with hegemonic norms. While *Beat the Devil* contains a sense of righteous and justified rage, its protagonist appears oblivious to the underhanded nature of hegemony. Decrying the government's claims that their marketized approach facilitated efficiency and international respect, he exclaims, 'Does it never occur to the great minds of British politics that there is a direct connection between honesty and popularity? Why is that idea so hard to grasp? Has no one in the current government ever met the bereaved?' (Hare 2020, 17). Although this complaint is nothing new, its central thesis is grounded in a liberal idealism and faith in reason that overestimates honesty's political currency and misdiagnoses how ideology exerts its power. While ideological falsehoods are partly designed to trick people into beliefs counter to their interests, their 'main function is neither to be believed or disbelieved, but to facilitate certain behaviours while constraining others. Sometimes this implies belief, but it need not do so' (Gilbert and Williams 2022, 43). While someone might intuit the dysfunction at the heart of healthcare privatization, the naturalization of the neoliberal market as having 'no alternative', combined with personal circumstances that offer a relatively comfortable life, might easily lead to complacent acceptance of the situation.

It is plain to see, of course, that such consent for neoliberalism is starting to fray as its contradictions intensify and living conditions worsen. However, for the most part, Hare does not address this phenomenon or the material factors affecting the wider world outside the political theater of Westminster or the White House. There is but one reference to the plight of the viral underclass, when Hare recalls how people in his social circle were annoyed with him for coming down with something they considered a disease for poor and minoritized people. As Hare dutifully reminds us, 'in England and Wales, you're four times as likely to die if you're black' (Hare 2020, 14), a short footnote that critic Andrzej Lukowsi suggests is 'crying out for deeper exploration'. Determined to simply recount the government's obvious failures, much of Hare's political discourse is 'determined not to stand the test of time' (Lukowski 2020) – an observation revealing Lukowski's sharp awareness of neoliberalism's hegemonic crisis. Many other critics offered similar views, praising Hare's poignant personal tale while politely bemoaning the lack of 'precise, needling critique one might have hoped for' (Davies 2020) and the fact that his 'character seems more angry about unprofessionalism than human suffering' (Saville 2020).

Given the exclusionary economics of the contemporary theater landscape, it should come as no surprise that one of the first major

COVID-19 plays amounted to what Lukowski describes as 'a posh middle-aged man playing a posh old man having a moan about the issues of the day' (Lukowski 2020). However, *Beat the Devil*'s lukewarm reception combined with the production of other, more incisive cultural outputs reflects wider political dynamics absent from the early days of the HIV/AIDS crisis. For example, despite the high profiles of Hare and Fiennes, the BBC rejected the opportunity to screen a television adaptation for a wider audience, citing lack of public interest. Quoted in the *Guardian*, Hare took umbrage with this explanation, stating: 'Anyone who saw Jack Thorne's film *Help*, about the care home crisis, will know that actually you can make very timely and urgent work about COVID-19 and people will want to watch it. So it's just complete nonsense' (Alberge 2021).

What Hare misses here is the fact that Thorne's pacy film – broadcast on the UK's Channel 4 in 2021 – tells stories that differ widely from his own in their classed dynamics and political overtones. *Help*'s protagonist, for example, a working-class care home worker in Liverpool, struggles to keep residents alive in the midst of pandemic chaos, plugging the gaps of a broken healthcare system in exchange for pitiful wages. Given the film's stark portrayal of the emotional and physical strain of such a poorly paid and thankless task, its success reveals an appetite for narratives reflecting the harsh reality of those at the sharp end of neoliberalism's cruelties – rather than a desire to listen to more well-worn complaints about those in power. More specifically, interest in the film reflects growing awareness of capitalism's crisis of care and social reproduction. While Hare talks of being lucky enough to enjoy the care of a devoted wife and a GP with the time to conduct twice-daily FaceTime consultations, the dying residents in *Help* represent the collateral damage of an alienating system designed to eke as much surplus value from broad swathes of the citizenry as possible. This impetus, however, also drains society of the labor resources it requires to reproduce itself and care for the sick, as shown in the sparsely staffed care home in *Help*. Indeed, lack of care resources is a key contradiction revealing capitalism's 'tendency to social-reproductive crisis' (Fraser and Jaeggi 2018, 35). While the nuclear-family model remains hegemonic, households are increasingly reliant on multiple earners' wages, reducing their capacity to fulfill caring responsibilities. At the same time, evermore threadbare welfare provisions and the 'corporate seizure of care homes from the public sector [...] has meant that the people being "cared for" in their own communities are often neglected' (The Care Collective 2020, 15). At some point, something has got to give.

Although current economic structures continue to privilege certain types of art, it would make sense that the broad appetite for alternative stories and consciousness-raising work might be greater now compared to the early years of the HIV/AIDS pandemic. While certain queer and classed constituencies faced quasi-apocalyptic prospects in the early years of the crisis, of course, the broader political context was such that capitalist liberal democracy appeared to have won its hegemonic battle against socialist alternatives. Neoliberal ideologues espoused the virtues of the free market and the promise of material gains through individual hard work – a narrative that spoke to the interests of the still relatively substantial middle classes. Today, the fundamental falsehoods of such promises are achingly clear and the crises more all-encompassing, creating an increasingly large contingent of politicized subjects disillusioned by neoliberalism's failures. So, despite the political limitations of Hare's play, some of the more experimental pandemic theater to grace London's major theaters recognized the potential to reach such audiences.

The Royal Court, for example, hosted a series of so-called Living Newspapers – shows comprising theatricalized news stories and features, 'including local and global perspectives, longer form pieces, a dating column, a cartoon of the week, a weather room, an agony aunt, your horoscopes, and more' (The Royal Court 2021). Performed in various spaces across the theater, including its backstage areas, the 'newspapers' were broadcast online to a much wider viewership. As well as commissioning highly political work addressing the issues of the day from a variety of counterhegemonic perspectives, the theater actively sought new and upcoming writers and performers to get involved. This approach reflects the ethos of the Federal Theater Project – an arts program established in the Depression-era US and upon which the Royal Court's Living Newspaper project was based. Established partly to mobilize unemployed artists, the project took inspiration from living newspapers staged in Europe and Bolshevik Russia, which were designed to inform illiterate workers about current affairs. Updated for modern audiences, the Royal Court's Living Newspapers were similarly geared toward social change and accessibility, offering inexpensive online admission and short, uncomplicated theatrical snippets covering topics from the government's pandemic failures to interconnected issues such as global heating and economic decline. In so doing, it used the COVID-19 crisis as a starting point with which 'to question what we really know, think and feel about our current unprecedented historical moment' (Marlowe 2020), undermining hegemonic narratives that emerge from a media ecology largely beholden to corporate interests.

Given the very different sociopolitical environment we find ourselves in now compared to the first few decades of the HIV/AIDS crisis, what might a politicized HIV/AIDS theater look like now and in the future? At this point, it is important to reiterate the fragility of progress in regard to HIV/AIDS treatments and outcomes. While it might be the case that the introduction of pharmaceuticals such as protease inhibitors has curbed transmission and death rates in certain parts of the world, this trajectory is vulnerable to setbacks and reversals. Take Greece, for example. Following the economic crash of 2008, the debt-ridden country was forced to further neoliberalize its economy at the behest of the 'troika' – the IMF, European Commission, and European Central Bank. As a result, Greece lost over 30% of its GDP and witnessed a steep deterioration in its healthcare infrastructures, losing its ability to provide quality care for people with HIV. Somewhat predictably, drug-related HIV infections in Greece rose by over 400% between 2010 and 2012 (The Care Collective 2020, 73), a figure that underlines the interconnectedness of the HIV/AIDS crisis with other social and economic crises. As a 2013 study of the spread of HIV in the US revealed, 'HIV infection is so closely enmeshed in conditions of poverty that it is [...] a pandemic of the poor', with the authors noting that ameliorative action such as substance abuse programs and humanitarian health interventions 'will mean nothing unless the barriers posed by racism, homophobia, stigmas and discrimination are lifted. Our best chance for reducing the health disparity [...] will be to address social and structural factors that underlie the HIV epidemic' (Pellowski et al. 2013, 12). Any project designed to tackle HIV/AIDS must, therefore, take a broader view of our conjunctural crises and the huge scale of the task at hand.

Several of the HIV/AIDS plays I have examined in this study recognize the far-reaching negative impacts of neoliberal alienation and crises of social reproduction – from Neil Watkins' assertion that we are all outsiders in need of joining forces to fight oppression, to Donja Love's critique of those audience members who are yet to take action to fight health injustice. What joins these works together is their interrogation of theater as a tool to drive change, mired as it often is within hegemonic structures and corporate interests. Disappointed or discontented with the genre's historical trajectory, HIV/AIDS playwrights are starting to undo some of its more conservative impulses and lay the groundwork to shift public consciousness surrounding the pandemic. Of course, as the twenty-first century progresses and political volatility likely increases across the globe, it remains to be seen how future HIV/AIDS playwrights will build on this key insight. Perhaps, as Prior declares at the very end of *Angels in America*, 'The Great Work Begins' (Kushner [1993] 2017, 290).

Bibliography

@DeanneChen. "@thenormalheart hit my conscious with a sledgehammer and demolished me into a sobbing mess. Pls learn more about HIV/AIDS: www.aids.gov." Twitter, July 11, 2011, 4:54 a.m. https://twitter.com/DeanneChen/status/90267696096215040.

@donlemon. "What an incredible show & cast. so emotional. I'm dehydrated from crying so much. wow. larry was there too." Twitter, May 25, 2011, 3:41 p.m. https://twitter.com/donlemon/status/73398279337021440.

Abdoh, Reza. 1996. "The Law of Remains." In *Plays for the End of the Century*, edited by Bonnie Maranca, 9–94. Baltimore, MD: Johns Hopkins University Press.

Abramowitz, Ben. 2019. "Pfizer, GSK Fight HIV with Immersive Theater (and Drugs)." Syneos Health Communications, September 17. https://syneoshealthcommunications.com/blog/pfizer-gsk-fight-hiv-with-immersive-theater-and-drugs.

Adler-Bolton, Beatrice, and Artie Vierkant. 2022. *Health Communism*. London: Verso.

Alberge, Dalya. 2021. "David Hare Furious at BBC after It Rejects His Covid Play, Starring Ralph Fiennes." *The Observer*, October 24. https://www.theguardian.com/culture/2021/oct/24/david-hare-furious-bbc-rejection-of-covid-play.

Altman, Lawrence K. 1981. "Rare Cancer Seen in 41 Homosexuals." *The New York Times*, July 3. https://www.nytimes.com/1981/07/03/us/rare-cancer-seen-in-41-homosexuals.html.

André, Kévin, Sylvain Bureau, Arthur Gautier, and Olivier Rubel. 2017. "Beyond the Opposition between Altruism and Self-Interest: Reciprocal Giving in Reward-Based Crowdfunding." *Journal of Business Ethics* 146 (2): 313–32. https://doi.org/10.1007/s10551-017-3652-x.

Andriote, John-Manuel. 1999. *Victory Deferred: How AIDS Changed Gay Life in America*. Chicago: University of Chicago Press.

Armengol, Josep M. 2001. "Gendering the Irish Land: Seamus Heaney's 'Act of Union.'" *Aedean* 23 (1): 7–26.

Armstrong, Martin. 2022. "Here's How Global GDP Has Changed over the Past 40 Years." World Economic Forum, October 20. https://www.weforum.org/agenda/2022/10/global-gdp-asia-economy/.

Artel, Sabrina. 1995. "At Breakneck Speed: Performing with Dar a Luz." *TDR* 39 (4): 72.

Arthur, Marc. 2021. "Nostalgia and Chronicity: Two Temporalities in the Restaging of AIDS." *Theatre Journal* 73 (1): 19–36.

"As Much as I Can." n.d. Harley & Company. Accessed April 17, 2023. https://www.harleyandcompany.com/as-much-as-i-can-1.

Balani, Sita. 2023. *Deadly and Slick: Sexual Modernity and the Making of Race*. London: Verso.

Barnes-McLain, Noreen. 1997. "Death and Desire: The Evolution of the AIDS Play." *Journal of Dramatic Theory and Criticism* 12 (1): 113–20.

Bechtel, Roger. 2001. "'A Painful Kind of Progress': The Benjaminian Dialectics of *Angels in America*." *Journal of Dramatic Theory and Criticism* 1 (16): 99–120.

Bell, Jonathan. 2018. "Between Private and Public: AIDS, Health Care Capitalism, and the Politics of Respectability in 1980s America." *Journal of American Studies* 1 (May): 1–25.

Benjamin, Walter. (1968) 2015. *Illuminations*. Edited by Hannah Arendt. Translated by Harry Zorn. London: Penguin.

Bennington-Castro, Joseph. 2020. "How AIDS Remained an Unspoken—but Deadly—Epidemic for Years." History, June 1. https://www.history.com/news/aids-epidemic-ronald-reagan.

Berger, Mark Alan. 2019. "'As Much as I Can' Blurs Reality with Fantasy." *Interview Magazine*, September 13. https://www.interviewmagazine.com/culture/as-much-as-i-can-sarah-hall-immersive-play-joes-pub.

Bersani, Leo. (1995) 2009. *Homos*. Cambridge, MA: Harvard University Press.

Billington, Michael. 2017. "*Angels in America* Review – Garfield and Lane Excel in Kushner's Surreal Epic." *The Guardian*, May 5. www.theguardian.com/stage/2017/may/05/angels-in-america-review-andrew-garfield-nathan-lane-tony-kushner.

Blakeley, Grace. 2019. *Stolen: How to Save the World from Financialisation*. London: Repeater Books.

Boerner, Heather. 2022. "Lack of Access to Resources Makes Black Folks More Vulnerable to HIV." *POZ*, February 7. https://www.poz.com/article/lack-access-resources-makes-black-folks-vulnerable-hiv.

Boeuf, Benjamin, Jessica Darveau, and Renaud Legoux. 2014. "Financing Creativity: Crowdfunding as a New Approach for Theatre Projects." *International Journal of Arts Management* 16 (3): 33–48.

Bottoms, Stephen. 2006. "Putting the Documentary into Documentary: An Unwelcome Corrective?" *The Drama Review* 50 (3): 56–68.

Bratton, Benjamin. 2021. *Revenge of the Real: Politics for a Post-Pandemic World*. London: Verso.

Breslauer, Jan. 1994. "'Sharing the Delirium' of AIDS: Theater: A New Collection of Predominantly Activist-Oriented Stage Works Illustrates 'the Division between First- and Second-Generation AIDS Plays', the Book's Editor Says. Six of the Seven Are by West Coast Writers." *Los Angeles Times*, May 21. https://www.latimes.com/archives/la-xpm-1994-05-21-ca-60416-story.html.

British Medical Association. 2020. "The Role of Private Outsourcing in the COVID-19 Response." https://www.bma.org.uk/media/2885/the-role-of-private-outsourcing-in-the-covid-19-response.pdf.

Brown, Wendy. 1995. *States of Injury: Power and Freedom in Late Modernity*. Princeton, NJ: Princeton University Press.

———. 2006. "American Nightmare: Neoliberalism, Neoconservatism, and De-Democratization." *Political Theory* 34 (6): 690–714.

———. 2019. *In the Ruins of Neoliberalism: The Rise of Antidemocratic Politics in the West*. New York: Columbia University Press.

Burns, William E. 2011. *Science in the Enlightenment: An Encyclopedia*. Santa Barbara, CA: Abc-Clio.

Butler, Isaac, and Dan Kois. 2018. *The World Only Spins Forward: The Ascent of Angels in America*. New York: Bloomsbury USA.

Byttebier, Stephanie. 2011. "'It Doesn't Count If It's Easy': Facing Pain, Mediating Identity in Tony Kushner's *Angels in America*." *Modern Drama* 54 (3): 287–309. https://doi.org/10.1353/mdr.2011.0033.

Campbell, Alyson. 2011. "From Bogeyman to Bison: A Herd-like Amnesia of HIV/AIDS in Theatre?" *Theatre Research International* 36 (3): 196–212.

Campbell, Alyson, and Dirk Gindt. 2018. *Viral Dramaturgies: HIV and AIDS in Performance in the Twenty-First Century*. Basingstoke: Palgrave Macmillan.

The Care Collective. 2020. *The Care Manifesto: The Politics of Interdependence*. London: Verso.

Carroll, Tamar W. 2015. *Mobilizing New York: AIDS, Antipoverty, and Feminist Activism*. Chapel Hill: University of North Carolina Press.

Central Office of Information for Department of Health. 1987. "AIDS Monolith." https://webarchive.nationalarchives.gov.uk/ukgwa/20230801151623/https:/www.nationalarchives.gov.uk/films/1979to2006/filmpage_aids.htm.

Cermatori, Joseph. 2020. "Radical Gesture and the Politics of Postdramatic Tragedy: Reza Abdoh's *The Law of Remains*." *Journal of Contemporary Drama in English* 8 (1): 127–42.

Ceron, Ella. 2023. "The Pay Gap for Single Women Is Getting Worse." *Time*, March 8. https://time.com/6260969/gender-pay-gap-single-women/.

Chacon, Alexi. 2022. "There's an Overlooked Multitude of Excellent HIV-Focused Plays." *The Body*, December 9. https://www.thebody.com/article/overlooked-multitude-excellent-hiv-focused-plays.

Chambers-Letson, Joshua. 2018. "Hovering in the Impasse: Reza Abdoh and the Uses of Blackness." Walker Art Center, May 29. https://walkerart.org/magazine/hovering-in-the-impasse-reza-abdoh-and-the-uses-of-blackness.

Chanan, Michael. 2022. *From Printing to Streaming: Cultural Production under Capitalism*. London: Pluto Press.

Chase, Marilyn. 1989. "Burroughs Wellcome Reaps Profits, Outrage from Its AIDS Drugs." *Wall Street Journal*, September 15.

Cheng, Jih-Fei. 2020. "AIDS, Women of Color Feminisms, Queer and Trans of Color Critiques, and the Crises of Knowledge Production." In *AIDS and the Distribution of Crises*, edited by Jih-Fei Cheng, Alexandra Juhasz, and Nishant Shahani, 76–92. Durham, NC: Duke University Press.

Cheng, Jih-Fei, Alexandra Juhasz, and Nishant Shahani, eds. 2020. *AIDS and the Distribution of Crises*. Durham, NC: Duke University Press.

Chitty, Christopher. 2020. *Sexual Hegemony: Statecraft, Sodomy, and Capital in the Rise of the World System*. Durham, NC: Duke University Press.

chloethefry. 2022. "Interview: Alexis Gregory – Riot Act." CentreStage, May 8. https://cfrycentrestage.wordpress.com/2022/05/08/interview-alexis-gregory-riot-act/.

Cifor, Marika. 2022. *Viral Cultures: Activist Archiving in the Age of AIDS*. Minneapolis: University of Minnesota Press.

Cockburn, Paul. 2017. "*5 Guys Chillin'*: 4 Star Review by Paul F Cockburn." Broadwaybaby.com, August 8. https://broadwaybaby.com/shows/5-guys-chillin/721397.

Cohen, Cathy J. 1999. *The Boundaries of Blackness: AIDS and the Breakdown of Black Politics*. Chicago: University of Chicago Press.

Cohen, Randy. 2019. "NEA Budget Losses." *National Arts Administration and Policy Publications Database*. Administration for the Arts. https://www.americansforthearts.org/by-program/reports-and-data/legislation-policy/naappd/nea-budget-losses.

Coulter, Colin. 2015. "Ireland under Austerity." In *Ireland under Austerity: Neoliberal Crisis, Neoliberal Solutions*, edited by Colin Coulter and Angela Nagle, 1–44. Manchester: Manchester University Press.

Crimp, Douglas. 2011. "Before Occupy: How AIDS Activists Seized Control of the FDA in 1988." *The Atlantic*, December 6. https://www.theatlantic.com/health/archive/2011/12/before-occupy-how-aids-activists-seized-control-of-the-fda-in-1988/249302/.

Curtis, Nick. 2021. "*The Normal Heart* Review: A Timely and Essential Revival." *The Standard*, October 1. https://www.standard.co.uk/culture/theatre/the-normal-heart-review-national-theatre-aids-b958259.html.

Darney, Peter. 2016. *5 Guys Chillin'*. London: Oberon.

Dasgupta, Gautam. 1994. "Body/Politic: The Ecstasies of Reza Abdoh." *Performing Arts Journal* 16 (3): 18–27.

Davies, Ava Wong. 2020. "Ralph Fiennes Stars in Slapdash and Heavy-Handed Covid Monologue 'Beat the Devil.'" *The Independent*, September 1. https://www.independent.co.uk/arts-entertainment/theatre-dance/reviews/beat-the-devil-review-ralph-fiennes-covid-19-plot-tickets-a9698301.html.

Dawson, Michael C., and Megan Ming Francis. 2015. "Black Politics and the Neoliberal Racial Order." *Public Culture* 28 (1): 23–62.

Dean, Jodi. 2019. *Comrade: An Essay on Political Belonging*. London: Verso.

Dean, Tim. 2009. *Unlimited Intimacy: Reflections on the Subculture of Barebacking*. Chicago: University of Chicago Press.

Delgado, Maria M., and Caridad Svich, eds. 2002. *Theatre in Crisis? Performance Manifestos for a New Century*. Manchester: Manchester University Press.

D'Emilio, John. 1993. "Capitalism and Gay Identity." In *The Lesbian and Gay Studies Reader*, edited by David M. Halperin, Henry Abelove, and Michele Aina Barale, 467–76. London: Routledge.

Dowden, Neil. 2018. "The Inheritance: An Engaging Epic about 21st Century Gay Identity." *Londonist*, October 19. https://londonist.com/london/on-stage/the-inheritance-noel-coward-theatre-review.

Drucker, Peter. 2015. *Warped: Gay Normality and Queer Anti-Capitalism*. Chicago: Haymarket Books.

Duggan, Lisa. 2003. *The Twilight of Equality? Neoliberalism, Cultural Politics, and the Attack on Democracy*. Boston: Beacon Press.

Edelman, Lee. 2004. *No Future: Queer Theory and the Death Drive*. Durham, NC: Duke University Press.

Farrier, Stephen. 2015. "Playing with Time: Gay Intergenerational Performance Work and the Productive Possibilities of Queer Temporalities." *Journal of Homosexuality* 62 (10): 1398–418.

Feingold, Michael. 1999. "Artaud You So." In *Reza Abdoh*, edited by Daniel Mufson, 104–7. Baltimore, MD: Johns Hopkins University Press.

Findlay, Cait. 2022. "Review of Alexis Gregory's *Riot Act*." *Diva Magazine*, February 3. https://diva-magazine.com/2022/02/03/review-riot-act-alexis-gregory/.

Fisher, Mark. 2014. *Ghosts of My Life: Writings on Depression, Hauntology and Lost Futures*. Hants: Zero Books.

Flynn, Paul. 2015. "Addicted to Chemsex: 'It's a Horror Story.'" *The Observer*, November 22. https://www.theguardian.com/world/2015/nov/22/addicted-to-chemsex-gay-drugs-film.

Foley, Barbara. 2018. "Intersectionality: A Marxist Critique." *Science & Society* 82 (2): 269–75.

Fordyce, Ehren. 2004. "This Is Home, This Isn't Home: Reza Abdoh's *Tight Right White*." *Modern Drama* 47 (2): 219–36.

Forster, E.M. (1910) 2012. *Howards End*. London: Penguin.

Foster, Roger. 2016. "Therapeutic Culture, Authenticity and Neo-Liberalism." *History of the Human Sciences* 29 (1): 99–116.

Framke, Caroline. 2018. "TV Review: 'Pose' on FX." *Variety*, May 30. https://variety.com/2018/tv/reviews/pose-fx-review-ryan-murphy-1202824492/.

Fraser, Nancy. 2017a. "From Progressive Neoliberalism to Trump—and Beyond." *American Affairs Journal*, November 20. http://americanaffairsjournal.org/2017/11/progressive-neoliberalism-trump-beyond.

———. 2017b. "Progressive Neoliberalism versus Reactionary Populism: A Hobson's Choice." In *The Great Regression*, edited by Heinrich Geiselberger, 40–48. Cambridge: Polity.

———. 2019. *The Old Is Dying and the New Cannot Be Born: From Progressive Neoliberalism to Trump and Beyond*. London: Verso.

———. 2022. *Cannibal Capitalism: How Our System Is Devouring Democracy, Care, and the Planet – and What We Can Do about It*. New York: Verso.

Fraser, Nancy, and Rahel Jaeggi. 2018. *Capitalism: A Conversation in Critical Theory*. Cambridge: Polity.

Free, Marcus, and Clare Scully. 2018. "The Run of Ourselves: Shame, Guilt and Confession in Post-Celtic Tiger Irish Media." *International Journal of Cultural Studies* 21 (3): 308–24.

Frosini, Fabio. 2019. "Time and Revolution in Gramsci's *Prison Notebooks*." In *Revisiting Gramsci's Notebooks*, edited by Francesca Antonini, Aaron Bernstein, Lorenzo Fusaro, and Robert Jackson, 125–40. Boston: Brill.

Fukuyama, Francis. 1989. "The End of History?" *The National Interest* 1 (16): 3–18.

Gallant, Paul. 2022. "Has British Iconoclast David Hoyle Unwittingly Turned Himself into an Icon?" *Xtra Magazine*, June 15. https://xtramagazine.com/culture/david-hoyle-icon-224981.

Garside, Emily. 2022. "Theatre Review: Alexis Gregory's *Riot Act* ★★★★★." *The Queer Review*, August 13. https://thequeerreview.com/2022/08/12/theatre-review-riot-act-digital-edition/.

Genter, Robert. 2017. "Removing the Mask of Sanity: McCarthyism and the Psychiatric–Confessional Foundations of the Cold War National Security State." *Journal of American Studies* 52 (04): 1066–94. https://doi.org/10.1017/s0021875817000950.

Gilbert, Jeremy. 2013. "What Kind of Thing Is 'Neoliberalism'?" *New Formations* 80–81: 7–22.

———. 2015. *Common Ground: Democracy and Collectivity in an Age of Individualism.* London: Pluto Press.

Gilbert, Jeremy, and Alex Williams. 2022. *Hegemony Now: How Big Tech and Wall Street Won the World (and How We Win It Back).* New York: Verso.

Gilson, D. 2015. "LOLZ with Hillz: Neoliberal Power Circuits in the Divahood of Hillary Clinton." *The Journal of Popular Culture* 48 (4): 627–38.

Gindt, Dirk. 2018. "National Performances of Crying: Neoliberal Sentimentality and the Cultural Commodification of HIV and AIDS in Sweden." In *Viral Dramaturgies: HIV and AIDS in Performance in the Twenty-First Century,* edited by Alyson Campbell and Dirk Gindt, 235–54. Cham, Switzerland: Palgrave Macmillan.

Graff, Torsten. 2001. "Gay Drama/Queer Performance." *American Studies* 46 (1): 11–25.

Gramsci, Antonio. 2003. *Selections from the Prison Notebooks of Antonio Gramsci.* Edited by Quintin Hoare and Geoffrey Nowell-Smith. New York: Lawrence and Wishart.

Grayson, Deborah, and Ben Little. 2017. "Conjunctural Analysis and the Crisis of Ideas." *Soundings* 65 (1): 59–75.

Greer, Stephen. 2018. *Queer Exceptions: Solo Performance in Neoliberal Times.* Manchester: Manchester University Press.

Haas, Astrid. 2011. *Stages of Agency: The Contributions of American Drama to the AIDS Discourse.* Heidelberg: Universitatsverlag Winter.

Hackworth, Jason R. 2012. *Faith Based: Religious Neoliberalism and the Politics of Welfare in the United States.* Athens: University of Georgia Press.

Hakim, Jamie. 2015. "We Need to Stop the Moral Panic around Chemsex." Open Democracy, December 1. https://www.opendemocracy.net/en/transformation/we-need-to-stop-moral-panic-around-chemsex/.

Hall, Nathaniel. 2019. "First Time." Crowdfunder UK. https://www.crowdfunder.co.uk/p/first-time-at-the-edinburgh-fringe-festival-2019.

Hall, Stuart. 1996. "New Ethnicities." In *Stuart Hall: Critical Dialogues in Cultural Studies,* edited by Kuan-Hsing Chen and David Morley, 441–9. London: Routledge.

———. 2011. "The Neoliberal Revolution." *Soundings* 48 (August): 9–28. https://doi.org/10.3898/136266211797146828.

———. 2017. "Stuart Hall: Gramsci and Us." Verso Books blog. https://www.versobooks.com/blogs/2448-stuart-hall-gramsci-and-us.

Hall, Stuart, and Doreen Massey. 2010. "Interpreting the Crisis." *Soundings* 44: 57–71.

Hall, Stuart, and Alan O'Shea. 2013. "Common-Sense Neoliberalism." *Soundings* 55: 9–25.

Hancock, Ange-Marie. 2004. *The Politics of Disgust.* New York: New York University Press.

Hannabach, Cathy. 2016. *Blood Cultures: Medicine, Media, and Militarisms*. New York: Palgrave Macmillan.

Haraway, Donna. 1988. "Situated Knowledges: The Science Question in Feminism and the Privilege of Partial Perspective." *Feminist Studies* 14 (3): 575–99.

Hare, David. 2020. *Beat the Devil*. London: Faber & Faber.

Harley & Company. 2019. "As Much as I Can: Short Film." June 29. https://youtu.be/QxVK0eyOoaA.

Harris, Gareth. 2022. "Public Body Arts Council England at Risk under New UK Government Review." *The Art Newspaper*, May 18. https://www.theartnewspaper.com/2022/05/18/public-body-arts-council-england-at-risk-under-new-uk-government-review.

Harvard College Library. n.d. "Collection: ACT UP Oral History Project Digital Collection, 2002–2015." Hollisarchives.lib.harvard.edu. Accessed December 14, 2022. https://hollisarchives.lib.harvard.edu/repositories/31/resources/6341.

Harvey, David. 2005. *A Brief History of Neoliberalism*. Oxford: Oxford University Press.

Harvie, Jen. 2013. *Fair Play: Art, Performance and Neoliberalism*. Basingstoke: Palgrave Macmillan.

Haslett, Tobi. n.d. "Blasted: On Reza Abdoh's *Tight Right White*." *Bidoun*. Accessed April 17, 2023. https://www.bidoun.org/articles/Blasted.

Heaney, Seamus. 2001. "Act of Union." In *North*. London: Faber and Faber, 24–28.

Heddon, Deirdre. 2008. *Autobiography and Performance*. Basingstoke: Palgrave Macmillan.

Helms, Jesse. 1987. "S.Amdt.963 to H.R.3058 – 100th Congress (1987–1988)." October 14. https://www.congress.gov/amendment/100th-congress/senate-amendment/963.

Hemming, Sarah. 2017. "*Angels in America*, National Theatre (Lyttelton), London — Astonishing, Madly Inventive." *Financial Times*, May 5. https://www.ft.com/content/6e8de008-3188-11e7-9555-23ef563ecf9a.

Hennessy, Rosemary. 1998. *Profit and Pleasure: Sexual Identities in Late Capitalism*. Ann Arbor, MI: Taylor and Francis.

Henwood, Doug. 2015. "What the Sharing Economy Takes." *The Nation*, January 27. https://www.thenation.com/article/archive/what-sharing-economy-takes/.

Hernandez, Robb. 2019. *Archiving an Epidemic: Art, AIDS, and the Queer Chicanx Avant-Garde*. New York: New York University Press.

Hickel, Jason. 2013. "Neoliberal Plague: AIDS and Global Capitalism." Africa at LSE, March 8. https://blogs.lse.ac.uk/africaatlse/2013/03/08/neoliberal-plague-aids-and-global-capitalism/.

Higgins, Charlotte. 2010. "Arts Funding Cut 30% in Spending Review." *The Guardian*, October 20. https://www.theguardian.com/politics/2010/oct/20/arts-cuts-spending-review-council.

HIV.gov. 2019. "PEPFAR." January 11. https://www.hiv.gov/federal-response/pepfar-global-aids/pepfar.

———. 2021. "U.S. Statistics." June 2. https://www.hiv.gov/hiv-basics/overview/data-and-trends/statistics.

———. 2022. "The Global HIV/AIDS Epidemic." August 3. https://www.hiv.gov/hiv-basics/overview/data-and-trends/global-statistics.

Hobbes, Michael. 2014. "Why Did AIDS Ravage the U.S. More Than Any Other Developed Country?" *The New Republic*, May 12. https://newrepublic.com/article/117691/aids-hit-united-states-harder-other-developed-countries-why.

Hochstrasser, Tim. 2017. "Live Theatre UK." Live Theatre UK, May 19. https://livetheatreuk.co.uk/2017/05/19/review-5-guys-chillin/.

Holden, Stephen. 1999. "Theatre in Review: *The Law of Remains*." In *Reza Abdoh*, edited by Daniel Mufson, 102–3. Baltimore, MD: Johns Hopkins University Press.

Holloway, John. 2010. *Crack Capitalism*. London: Pluto Press.

Howard, Jane. 2012. "Fringe Review: *The Year of Magical Wanking*." No Plain Jane, March 5. http://noplain.wordpress.com/2012/03/05/fringe-review-the-year-of-magical-wanking.

Hughes, Holly, and David Román. 1998. *O Solo Homo: The New Queer Performance*. New York: Grove Press.

The Inheritance Play. 2019a. "Happy Birthday, Hillary Clinton! Jasper (Kyle Harris) Is with You Now and Forever." October 1. http://facebook.com/inheritanceplay/photos/a.379238832594963/711130232739153/?type=3&theater.

———. 2019b. "Each Has a Story Aching to Come Out… First Preview, Part One: 9.27.19. Share Your Story with Us: Https://TheInheritancePlay.com/Community." November 6. http://www.facebook.com/inheritanceplay/videos/458921308046323/.

———. n.d. "Community." Inheritance Broadway. Accessed November 6, 2019. http://theinheritanceplay.com/community.

———. n.d. "The Inheritance Play | Home | Official Broadway Site." Inheritance Broadway. Accessed November 6, 2019. http://theinheritanceplay.com.

Jaymes, Paul. 2007a. "David Hoyle – Live – Magazine – Issue: HIV Ünt AIDS. Part 3." September 3. www.youtube.com/watch?v=vYxxJxZwLSA.

———. 2007b. "David Hoyle – Live – Magazine – HIV Ünt AIDS Issue – Part 1." September 10. https://www.youtube.com/watch?v=Oz_fm1hUZVo.

———. 2007c. "David Hoyle – Live – Magazine – Issue: HIV Ünt AIDS. Part 2." September 10. https://www.youtube.com/watch?v=CxaurGhvmRw.

Johnson, Dominic. 2013. *Pleading in Blood: The Art and Performances of Ron Athey*. Bristol: Intellect.

Jones, Jason. 2018. "Review | 'Riot Act' – a New Verbatim Theatre Piece by Alexis Gregory." *Attitude*, August 1. https://www.attitude.co.uk/culture/film-tv/review-riot-act-a-new-verbatim-theatre-piece-by-alexis-gregory-296645/.

Jones, Rhodessa. 1998. "Deep in the Night." *Journal of Medical Humanities* 19 (2/3): 181–96.

Jones, Therese. 1994. *Sharing the Delirium*. Portsmouth, NH: Heinemann.

Jones, Wendell, and David Stanley. 1994. "AIDS! The Musical!" In *Sharing the Delirium: Second Generation AIDS Plays and Performances*, edited by Therese Jones. Portsmouth, NH: Heinemann, 207–63.

Joseph, Miranda. 2002. *Against the Romance of Community*. Minneapolis: University of Minnesota Press.

Juntunen, Jacob. 2016. *Mainstream AIDS Theatre, the Media, and Gay Civil Rights: Making the Radical Palatable*. Abingdon: Routledge.

Kanai, Akane, and Rosalind Gill. 2020. "Woke? Affect, Neoliberalism, Marginalised Identities and Consumer Culture." *New Formations* 102: 10–27. https://doi.org/10.3898/newf:102.01.2020.

Kickstarter. 2023. "Kickstarter Stats." Kickstarter, April 21. https://www.kickstarter.com/help/stats.

Kitchener, Shaun. n.d. "'Positive' at the Edinburgh Fringe." Kickstarter. Accessed April 21, 2023. https://www.kickstarter.com/projects/1839032474/positive-at-the-edinburgh-fringe/community.

Kramer, Larry. 1997. "Sex and Sensibility." *The Advocate*.

———. 2011. *The Normal Heart*. London: Nick Hern Books.

———. 2020. "March 27, 1983: 1,112 and Counting." *Los Angeles Blade*, May 27. https://www.losangelesblade.com/2020/05/27/march-27-1983-1112-and-counting/.

Kundnani, Arun. 2021. "The Racial Constitution of Neoliberalism." *Race & Class* 63 (1): 51–69.

Kushner, Tony. (1993) 2017. *Angels in America: A Gay Fantasia on National Themes*. London: Nick Hern Books.

Kushnir, Andrew, Paul Dunn, and Damien Atkins. 2018. *The Gay Heritage Project*. Toronto: Playwrights Canada Press.

Langley, Paul, and Andrew Leyshon. 2017. "Capitalizing on the Crowd: The Monetary and Financial Ecologies of Crowdfunding." *Environment and Planning A* 49 (5): 1019–39. https://doi.org/10.1177/0308518x16687556.

Leeming, David. 2006. "Wakan Tanka." In *The Oxford Companion to World Mythology*, 399. Oxford: Oxford University Press.

Levin, Sam. 2019. "'A Critical Point in History': How Trump's Attack on LGBT Rights Is Escalating." *The Guardian*, September 3. http://www.theguardian.com/world/2019/sep/03/trump-attack-lgbt-rights-supreme-court.

Levitow, Roberta. 2002. "Some Words About the Theatre Today." *Theatre in Crisis? Performance Manifestos for a New Century*, edited by Maria M. Delgado and Caridad Svich. Manchester: Manchester University Press, 25–30.

Long, Thomas L. 2005. *AIDS and American Apocalypticism: The Cultural Semiotics of an Epidemic*. New York: State University of New York Press.

Lopez, Matthew. 2018. *The Inheritance*. London: Faber and Faber.

Love, Donja R. 2022. *One in Two*. New York: Dramatists Play Service.

Lukowski, Andrzej. 2020. "'Beat the Devil' by David Hare Is a Fiery Covid Monologue Performed by Ralph Fiennes." *Time Out*, September 3. https://www.timeout.com/london/theatre/beat-the-devil-is-a-fiery-covid-monologue-performed-by-ralph-fiennes.

Luxton, Meg. 2010. "Doing Neoliberalism: Perverse Individualism in Personal Life." In *Neoliberalism and Everyday Life*, edited by Susan Braedley and Meg Luxton, 163–83. Montreal: McGill-Queen's University Press.

Magnuson, Joel. 2018. *Financing the Apocalypse: Drivers for Economic and Political Instability*. Cham, Switzerland: Palgrave Macmillan.

Mahase, Elisabeth. 2022. "NHS Outsourcing to Private Providers Is Associated with Rise in Treatable Deaths, Study Shows." *BMJ*, June.30: 377. https://doi.org/10.1136/bmj.o1612.

Marcuse, Herbert. (1964) 2002. *One-Dimensional Man*. London: Routledge.

Marlowe, Sam. 2020. "*Living Newspaper* Is Defiant, Energised and Embracing the Spirit of Immediacy and Provocation." Inews, December 17. https://inews.co.uk/culture/arts/living-newspaper-royal-court-review-defiant-energised-798932.

Marowitz, Charles. 1999. "Los Angeles in Review: *Bogeyman*." In *Reza Abdoh*, edited by Daniel Mufson, 99–101. Baltimore, MD: Johns Hopkins University Press.

Martin, James. 2022. *Hegemony*. Cambridge: Polity.

Marx, Karl. 2013. *Capital: A Critical Analysis of Capitalist Production*. Ware, Hertfordshire: Wordsworth Editions.

Mauss, Marcel. (1925) 1990. *The Gift: The Form and Reason for Exchange in Archaic Societies*. London: Routledge.

Mc, Philly. 2011. "The Year of Magical Wanking." https://fundit.ie/project/the-year-of-magical-wanking.

McNally, David. 1999. "The Present as History: Thoughts on Capitalism at the Millennium." *Monthly Review* 51 (3): 134.

Mead, Rebecca. 2019. "How Matthew Lopez Transformed 'Howards End' into an Epic Play about Gay Life." *The New Yorker*, August 29. https://www.newyorker.com/magazine/2019/09/09/how-matthew-lopez-transformed-howards-end-into-an-epic-play-about-gay-life.

Michaeli, Inna. 2017. "Self-Care: An Act of Political Warfare or a Neoliberal Trap?" *Development* 60 (1–2): 50–56.

Milazzo, Franco. 2011. "Interview: David Hoyle 'Philosopher King of Cabaret.'" *Londonist*, August 5. http://londonist.com/2011/08/interview-david-hoyle.

Miller, Tim. 1994. "My Queer Body." In *Sharing the Delirium: Second Generation AIDS Plays and Performances*, edited by Therese Jones, 309–36. Portsmouth, NH: Heinemann.

———. 2002. *Body Blows: Six Performances*. Madison: University of Wisconsin Press.

Miller, Tim, and David Román. 1995. "Preaching to the Converted." *Theatre Journal* 47 (2): 169–88.

Mineo, Liz. 2021. "Racial Wealth Gap May Be a Key to Other Inequities." *Harvard Gazette*, June 3. https://news.harvard.edu/gazette/story/2021/06/racial-wealth-gap-may-be-a-key-to-other-inequities/.

Mirowski, Philip. 2014. *Never Let a Serious Crisis Go to Waste: How Neoliberalism Survived the Financial Meltdown*. London: Verso.

Mullin, Brian. 2021. "'It's a Sin' Is a Transatlantic Hit. But It Repeats Tired AIDS Crisis Tropes." *Los Angeles Times*, February 23. https://www.latimes.com/entertainment-arts/tv/story/2021-02-23/its-a-sin-failures-of-hiv-representation.

Muñoz, José Esteban. 1999. *Disidentifications: Queers of Color and the Performance of Politics*. Minneapolis: University of Minnesota Press.

National Endowment for the Arts. 2021. "National Endowment for the Arts Supports the Arts with over $27.5 Million in Awards in First Round of FY2021 Funding." February 4. https://www.arts.gov/news/press-releases/2021/national-endowment-arts-supports-arts-over-275-million-awards-first-round-fy2021-funding.

National Theatre. 2017. *Angels in America* Program.

———. 2021. "Theatre and Activism: Larry Kramer's *The Normal Heart* and the 1980s AIDS Crisis." September 10. https://www.youtube.com/watch?v=cNFIrbl73Vg.

New York Times. 1996. "Text of President Clinton's Announcement on Welfare Legislation." August 1. https://www.proquest.com/blogs-podcasts-websites/text-president-clintons-announcement-on-welfare/docview/2237621289/se-2.

NewMagazine. 2007. "David Hoyle's Magazine. HIV Unt AIDS. ULI 01." October 20. https://www.youtube.com/watch?v=UJKWOqmuBQo.

O'Brien, Cormac. 2013. "Performing POZ: Irish Theatre, HIV Stigma, and 'Post-AIDS' Identities." *Irish University Review* 43 (1): 74–85.

O'Brien, Michelle. 2021. "Trans Work." In *Transgender Marxism*, edited by Jules Joanne Gleeson and Elle O'Rourke, 47–61. London: Pluto Press.

O'Neill, Edward R. 2007. "The M-m-Mama of Us All: Divas and the Cultural Logic of Late Ca(M)Pitalism." *Camera Obscura: Feminism, Culture, and Media Studies* 22 (2): 11–37.

Oliver, Daniel. 2014. "You're Funnier When You're Angry': Affirmation, Responsibility and Commitment in David Hoyle's Live Performance Practice." *Performance Research* 19 (2): 109–15.

Patton, Cindy. 1985. *Sex & Germs: The Politics of AIDS*. Montreal: Black Rose Books.

Pearl, Monica B. 2013. *AIDS Literature and Gay Identity: The Literature of Loss*. Abingdon: Routledge.

Pellowski, Jennifer A., Seth C. Kalichman, Karen A. Matthews, and Nancy Adler. 2013. "A Pandemic of the Poor: Social Disadvantage and the U.S. HIV Epidemic." *American Psychologist* 68 (4): 197–209.

Penney, James. 2014. *After Queer Theory: The Limits of Sexual Politics*. London: Pluto Press.

Petro, Anthony M. 2015. *After the Wrath of God: AIDS, Sexuality, and American Religion*. Oxford: Oxford University Press.

Philpott, Lachlan. 2010. *Bison/Closer*. Brisbane: Playlab Press.

Pisani, Elizabeth. 2008. *The Wisdom of Whores: Bureaucrats, Brothels, and the Business of AIDS*. New York: W. W. Norton.

Pomo Afro Homos. 2018. "Dark Fruit." In *Staging Gay Lives: An Anthology of Contemporary Gay Theater*, edited by John M. Clum, 319–43. New York: Routledge.

Purdy, Jedediah. 2014. "The Accidental Neoliberal." *N+1*, March 25. https://www.nplusonemag.com/issue-19/politics/the-accidental-neoliberal/.

Race, Kane. 2009. *Pleasure Consuming Medicine: The Queer Politics of Drugs*. Durham, NC: Duke University Press.

———. 2017. *The Gay Science*. Abingdon: Routledge.

Ralf, David. 2016. "Review: 5 Guys Chillin' at King's Head Theatre." *Exeunt Magazine*, February 15, 2016. https://exeuntmagazine.com/reviews/review-5-guys-chillin-at-kings-head-theatre/.

Reagan, Ronald. 1981. *America's New Beginning: A Program for Economic Recovery*. White House, Office of the Press Secretary. https://books.google.co.uk/books?id=K-XQAAAAMAAJ&printsec=.

Reed, Christopher A., Jonathan Livingston, Ariel Williams, Sherry C. Eaton, Leslie C. Brinson, Dwayne T. Brandon, and Grayson Chappell. 2015. "The Exploration of Theater as an Innovative Tool to Improve HIV Rates among Black Men." *Journal of Black Sexuality and Relationships* 1 (3): 75–96.

Rich, Frank. 1985. "Theater: 'The Normal Heart', by Larry Kramer." *The New York Times*, April 22. https://www.nytimes.com/1985/04/22/theater/theater-the-normal-heart-by-larry-kramer.html.

Roach, Tom. 2015. "Becoming Fungible." *Qui Parle* 23 (2): 55–87.

Rofes, Eric. 1998. *Dry Bones Breathe: Gay Men Creating Post-AIDS Identities and Cultures*. New York: Haworth Press.

Román, David. 1992. "Bogeyman." *Theatre Journal* 44 (3): 395.

———. 1998. *Acts of Intervention: Performance, Gay Culture, and AIDS*. Bloomington: Indiana University Press.

Rooney, David. 2018. "'Angels in America': Theater Review." *The Hollywood Reporter*, March 25. https://www.hollywoodreporter.com/news/general-news/angels-america-theater-review-1097127/.

Rosen, Rebecca J. 2012. "Kickstarter Expects to Provide More Funding than the National Endowment for the Arts This Year." *The Atlantic*, February 24. https://www.theatlantic.com/technology/archive/2012/02/kickstarter-expects-to-provide-more-funding-than-the-national-endowment-for-the-arts-this-year/253573/.

The Royal Court. 2021. "Living Newspaper Editions." https://royalcourttheatre.com/living-newspaper/.

Royles, Dan. 2020. *To Make the Wounded Whole: The African American Struggle against HIV/AIDS*. Chapel Hill: University of North Carolina Press.

Rudnick, Paul. 2010. "The Most Fabulous Story Ever Told." In *The Collected Plays of Paul Rudnick*, 135–246. New York: It Books.

Sackur, Leila. 2019. "Why We Should Question the 'Self-Care' of *Queer Eye*." *Dazed*, November 13. http://www.dazeddigital.com/beauty/soul/article/46797/1/queer-eye-self-care-fab-five-makeover-reality-tv-netflix.

Sanchez, Charles. 2019. "Immersive Theatre Production on Black Gay Men and HIV Gets Major New York City Run." *The Body*, September 19. https://www.thebody.com/article/black-lgbt-southern-hiv-conference-finds-new-home.

Sandoval-Sánchez, Alberto. 1999. *José, Can You See? Latinos on and off Broadway*. Madison: University of Wisconsin Press.

Sandset, Tony. 2019. "'HIV Both Starts and Stops with Me': Configuring the Neoliberal Sexual Actor in HIV Prevention." *Sexuality & Culture* 23 (2): 657–73. https://doi.org/10.1007/s12119-018-09584-1.

Saville, Alice. 2020. "Beat the Devil – Ralph Fiennes Stars in David Hare's Covid Monologue." *Financial Times*, September 2. https://www.ft.com/content/22cca05e-72c6-4ac6-9831-021d26537fcb.

Savran, David. 1995. "Ambivalence, Utopia, and a Queer Sort of Materialism: How 'Angels in America' Reconstructs the Nation." *Theatre Journal* 47 (2): 207–27. https://doi.org/10.2307/3208484.

Schulman, Sarah. 2021a. *Let the Record Show: A Political History of ACT UP New York, 1987–1993*. London: Picador.

———. 2021b. "What ACT UP's Successes Can Teach Today's Protest Movements." *The Guardian*, June 8. https://www.theguardian.com/commentisfree/2021/jun/08/act-up-protest-movements-us-direct-action.

Schulze, Daniel. 2017. *Authenticity in Contemporary Theatre and Performance: Make It Real*. London: Bloomsbury Methuen Drama.

Selman, Chris. 2022. "Nathaniel Hall's *First Time* Is an Utterly Essential Piece of Queer Theatre." *Gay Times*, February 11. https://www.gaytimes.co.uk/culture/nathaniel-halls-first-time-is-an-utterly-essential-piece-of-queer-theatre-review/.

Seymour, Richard. 2019. *The Twittering Machine*. London: Indigo.

Shanks, Gwyneth. 2018. "Patrick Scully on Performance, Protest, and Queer Politics." Walker Art Center. https://walkerart.org/magazine/when-your-friends-are-dying-you-damn-well-better-be-paying-attention-patrick-scully-on-performance-protest-and-queer-politics/.

Shenton, Mark. 2017. "*Angels in America* Review at the Lyttleton, National Theatre, London – 'Super-Sized.'" *The Stage*, May 5. www.thestage.co.uk/reviews/2017/angels-in-america-review-at-the-lyttelton-national-theatre-london.

Soch, Adam. 2016. "BOGEYMAN (1991) – Los Angeles – Created and Directed by Reza Abdoh." Vimeo, February 26. https://vimeo.com/156807754.

Somers-Willett, Susan. 2009. *The Cultural Politics of Slam Poetry: Race, Identity, and the Performance of Popular Verse in America*. Ann Arbor: University of Michigan Press.

Span, Paula, and Carla Hall. 1990. "Rejected! Portraits of the Performers the NEA Refused to Fund." *Washington Post*, January 2. https://www.washingtonpost.com/archive/lifestyle/style/1990/07/08/rejected-portraits-of-the-performers-the-nea-refused-to-fund/33481057-bf3d-4475-80a3-1d7cda452d33/.

Stamm, Laura. 2020. "Pose and HIV/AIDS." *TSQ: Transgender Studies Quarterly* 7 (4): 615–24.

Stayton, Richard. 2003. "The Next Life: 'Angels in America' Comes to HBO with Big Stars and Renewed Relevance." *Los Angeles Times*, November 30.

Steger, Manfred B., and Ravi K. Roy. 2010. *Neoliberalism: A Very Short Introduction*. Oxford: Oxford University Press.

Stuart, David. 2016. "Foreword." In Peter Darney, *5 Guys Chillin'*. London: Oberon.

Sukthankar, Ashwini. 1992. "Tim Miller Bares Queer Body in Original Stage Performance." *The Crimson*. http://www.thecrimson.com/article/1992/10/8/tim-miller-bares-queer-body-in.

Sullivan, Andrew. 1996. "When Plagues End." *The New York Times*, November 10. https://www.nytimes.com/1996/11/10/magazine/when-plagues-end.html.

Svich, Caridad. 2002. "Theatre in Crisis? Living Memory in an Unstable Time." In *Theatre in Crisis? Performance Manifestos for a New Century*, edited by Maria M. Delgado and Caridad Svich, 15–19. Manchester: Manchester University Press.

Táíwò, Olúfémi O. 2022. *Elite Capture: How the Powerful Took over Identity Politics (and Everything Else)*. London: Pluto Press.

Thrasher, Steven W. 2018. "Why Is *Angels in America* Still the Most Prominent Story Being Told about AIDS?" *BuzzFeed News*, March 25. https://www.buzzfeednews.com/article/steventhrasher/angels-in-america.

———. 2022. *The Viral Underclass*. New York: Celadon Books.

Trueman, Matt. 2018. "London Theater Review: 'The Inheritance.'" *Variety*, March 29. https://variety.com/2018/legit/reviews/the-inheritance-review-play-1202739184/.

Tyler, Imogen. 2020. *Stigma: The Machinery of Inequality*. London: Zed Books.

Valocchi, Stephen M. 2020. *Capitalisms and Gay Identities*. New York: Routledge.

Vile, Gareth K. 2016. "5 Guys Chillin'." *The List*, August 25. https://edinburghfestival.list.co.uk/article/84002-5-guys-chillin/.

Visser, Dirk. 2020. "Countering the Plague: AIDS Theatre as a Site of Memory." In *Literary and Visual Representations of HIV/AIDS: Forty Years Later*, edited by Aimee Pozorski, Jennifer J. Lavoie, and Christine J. Cynn. Lanham, MD: Lexington Books, 13–28.

Visual AIDS. 2013. "As We Canonize Certain Producers of Culture We Are Closing Space for a Complication of Narratives." December 10. https://visualaids.org/blog/as-we-canonize-certain-producers-of-culture-we-are-closing-space-for-a-comp.

Watkins, Neil. 2012. "The Year of Magical Wanking." In *The Oberon Anthology of Contemporary Irish Plays*, edited by Thomas Conway. London: Oberon.

Watney, Simon. 1997. *Policing Desire: Pornography, AIDS, and the Media*. London: Cassell.

West, Isaac. 2012. "Reviving Rage." *Quarterly Journal of Speech* 98 (1): 97–102.

Westerling, Kalle. 2018. "Mainstream Aids Theatre, the Media, and Gay Civil Rights: Making the Radical Palatable by Jacob Juntunen." *Theatre Journal* 70 (1): 127–28.

Williams, Raymond. 1989. *Marxism and Literature*. Oxford: Oxford University Press.

———. 2005. "Notes on Marxism in Britain since 1945." In *Culture and Materialism*, 261–81. London: Verso.

World Health Organization. 2020. "HIV/AIDS." https://www.who.int/data/gho/data/themes/hiv-aids.

Zimmerman, Guy. 2017. "The Captain in LA: Reza Abdoh's Bricolage and the Rise of Neoliberalism." *Theatre Journal* 69 (1): 61–79.

Index